# The Clinician's Thesaurus

A Guidebook for Wording Psychological Reports and Other Evaluations

Second Edition, Revised and Expanded

Edward L. Zuckerman, Ph. D.

Licensed Psychologist, Specialization in Clinical Psychology

Adjunct Associate Professor, Carnegie Mellon University

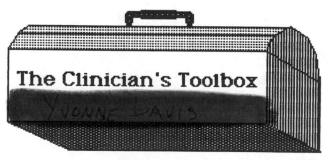

The Clinician's Toolbox

™

# Dedication

To my beloved daughter Molly.
This is what I was doing all those nights I was not with you.

ISBN 0-9622281-2-5                OCLC # 20591234

Copies of this book are available from the distributor you purchased from:

If you are unable to purchase from the above source the publisher will supply copies for $23.50 (which includes postage and handling) until at least the end of 1992. Bookstores pay postage but receive a discount of 25% from the list price of $19.95. Discounts for larger quantities are available; please write for details.

This book is available at significant discounts for bulk purchaser for educational uses, business gifts, and premiums. Specialized editions can also be created to meet specific needs; please contact the publisher.

The Clinician's Toolbox™ Series, which now includes *The Paper Office* (see last pages)

is published by

*Three Wishes Press*
Post Office Box 81033, Pittsburgh, PA 15217
(412) 521-1057 - Phone or Fax

The Clinician's Toolbox is a registered trademark and may not be copied or used without permission of the Publisher.

This book was created on a Apple Macintosh SE computer and a Hewlett Packard DeskWriter printer and is mainly set in their Times font.
Printed and bound in the United States of America by Bookcrafters
9 8 7 6 5 4 3

# 1. Introduction

If you create psychological documents such as Psychological or Psychiatric Evaluations, Progress Reports, Treatment Summaries, Testing-based Reports, Assessments, Intakes, Psychosocial Narratives, Staffing Reports, summaries of Interviews, or similar studies *The Clinician's Thesaurus* can make your work easier at the same time as it makes your reports better.

It is designed to assist you in writing inventive, tailored, fresh reports. The use of even five percent of the words and phrases collected here for any aspect of your observations will enhance the clarity, precision and vividness of your reports. And it can assist you in other ways as well:

• It is organized so that you can do a Mental Status Examination using its sequence and sampling from the questions offered.

• It can serve as a guide to organize your thoughts when writing or dictating reports to ensure that you have addressed all the topics of relevance.

• It can suggest behavioral observations to individualize and personalize a report or description.

• It can stimulate your recall of client characteristics (We all can recall more with the prompting of our memories).

• It can help to replace the drudgery of creating a narrative with playfulness, spontaneity, and serendipity.

• Because of its behavioral and observational bent and its gathering of clinically descriptive terms it is suitable for any clinical orientation or evaluation purpose.

To use *The Clinician's Thesaurus* most efficiently please understand that it is organized into five parts corresponding to the *sequence of constructing a report*. The first part contains two collections of questions which can be used to structure the interview with the patient. There are the traditional **Mental Status Questions** (and variations on them) for eliciting aspects of mental, cognitive, and emotional functioning of concern to the clinician. Then, if the clinician wishes to narrow the focus of the interview by following up on areas of clinical concern the second section contains questions designed to elicit information about specific **Symptomatic Behaviors**.

The rest of *The Clinician's Thesaurus* consists of four parts designed to serve as a guide to writing or dictating the actual report.

• First are the required contents of the **Introduction** to any report, the **Background** of the patient, **Reason for Referral**, and aspects of his or her **History**.

• Next are the standard areas of **Behavioral Observations** of the patient, and his or her **Interpersonal Behaviors** noted during the interview, including characteristics of **Speech** and **Affect**.

• The third part's sections provide many standard statements for use in describing **Normal** and **Abnormal Mental Statuses**, the common descriptors for reporting abnormal and **Symptomatic Behaviors**, an outline for DSM III **Diagnoses**, areas for **Recommendations** and ways of **Closing** the report.

• The fourth part offers sections containing standard statements for reporting evaluations of other

# Introduction

aspects of the patient's functioning: **Social** and interpersonal interactions, **Activities of Daily Living, Vocational** performance, **Recreational** pursuits, and other dimensions clinicians are often asked to evaluate. Then there is a section on commonly used descriptors for each type of **Personality** or character and, lastly, a list of **References** to the research on mental status examinations.

*The Clinician's Thesaurus* is, very simply, a tool to assist the already competent professional report writer in carrying out his or her tasks. Therefore it is not a textbook or treatise on "How to Write a Psychological Report" nor on clinical interviewing. Nor is it a set of psychological tests' interpretation statements as I have assumed that the reader is already well versed in these sophisticated clinical skills.

I must clearly acknowledge my debt to my colleagues from whose clearest thinking and best writing I have borrowed liberally to fill these pages. There are more than a hundred of you who have furnished the more than six thousand reports from which I have culled the 17,000 or so unduplicated wordings incorporated here. Although you are too numerous to credit please accept my gratitude and appreciation. While I have borrowed many of the words and phrases, I alone am responsible for the organization of *The Clinician's Thesaurus,* whatever its merits or limitations.

As you use *The Clinician's Thesaurus* you may find it valuable to underline, or highlight in color, particular words or phrases which best suit your style of writing or dictation and those most relevant to your own practice and setting. You may find it practical to use paperclips or to glue on tabs to more quickly find sections of the book. Space is purposely left blank so that you can add notes, comments and, especially, suggestions.

In this, the revised version of the second edition of *The Clinician's Thesaurus,* there is an additonal two percent more content than the earklier second edition which, in turn, expanded the first edition's content by about twent-five percent and added several tools useful to the report writer. I intend to keep this book in print at least until 1992 and would greatly value your ideas about how to make it even more useful to us clinicians. If you have suggestions or make additions to your copy please send me a photoccopy of those pages. If your suggestions are substantial and adopted into the next editon I will send you both a free copy and my sincerest thanks.

Edward Zuckerman
August 3, 1990
Pittsburgh, Pennsylvania

# 1. Table of Contents

**Notes**

# 3. General Notes

## 3.1 Descriptors:

The terms or descriptors offered in *The Clinician's Thesaurus* are arranged as either:
> a **Paragraph** of words and phrases having no ordering principle but simply often used together, or
> a **Spectrum** of words indicated by this sign (<->) and organized by either
>> - increasing intensity of the trait or behavior described or
>> - moving from "unhealthy" toward "healthy"
> a **Column** of quite similar but not identical terms which provide a cluster from which to select shadings of meaning. Where the first word is **Capitalized** it is the standard term used by clinicians for that cluster.

The terms offered are only rarely defined here. You may find a specialized dictionary useful such as Hinsie and Campbell (1970).

Words in **quotation marks** (" ") are slang or inappropriate in a professional report but are self-descriptors frequently offered by persons being evaluated and are placed under appropriate headings to assist the clinician unfamiliar with such phrasings in understanding their meanings.

Words often used in the evaluations of children but not adults are listed at the end of each section where they apply and are indicated by **For a Child:**

Commonly used acronyms are indicated by underlining the initial letters of the longer wording. For example, Activities of Daily Living.

The phrasings offered here are standard American English usage and conventional language.

## 3.2 Forms of Language:

For compactness and simplicity, adjectives, adverbs and nouns are sometimes mixed in a list.

The pronoun forms used here, while perhaps unfamiliar, are designed to lessen the harmful sexist associations and implications which are well documented to exist in this field. If, at times, pronouns of a single gender are employed that phrasing is for simplicity and should not be taken to imply any association of gender with disorder.

## 3.3 Attributions:

The psychologist, psychiatrist, social worker, nurse, therapist, counselor, clinician, behavior specialist, educator, teacher, advisor, interviewer, examiner, writer, reporter, respondent ...

can be said to report, offer, observe, document, note, relate, record, state, summarize ...

about the patient, client, claimant, resident, student, subject, individual, person, citizen, man, woman, child, adult. Boy or girl and use of a first or given name is acceptable only for children. Use Mr./Ms./Mrs./Dr./Esq. and other titles only if relevant.

He or she can be said to report, allege, submit, describe, claim, concede, indicate, maintain, attest to, mention, tell me, certify, state, offer, evidence, view, register, speak of, deny, disclaim, etc. Also acceptable is "was found to ...", and "appeared to be ...."

## 3.4 The Format used in this document is:

| | | |
|---|---|---|
| **1.** | **Section** | **14 Point Times Bold** |
| 1.1. | Heading | 14 Point Times |
| | Sub-heading | 12 POINT TIMES, SMALL CAPITALS |
| | Sub-sub-heading | *14 Point Italic* |
| | Sub-sub-heading | *12 Point Italic* |
| | Sub-sub-sub-heading | *12 Point Italic Underlined* |

## 3.5 White Spaces in the text:

Blank space is provided so you may customize the entries with your favorite phrases and statements. (I would be grateful for and attentive to your suggestions and improvements. If they are very useful I will send you a free copy of the next revision of *The Clinician's Thesaurus.* ELZ)

## 3.6 General notes on report writing:

Most agencies seem to prefer reports with:
a generous number of specific behavioral *observations*,
*example*s of symptomatic behaviors (as opposed to inferences and conclusions) and
many specific practical (those implementable in the client's current setting) *recommendations*.

Because of concerns with test security and copyrights do not repeat the questions from standardized tests or the mental status questions in your reports but only the responses received.

In reporting responses to objective questions it is clearer to the reader if you underline the erroneous responses, as for example on serial sevens: 93, 84, 77, 70, 62.

Avoid the use of acronyms, abbreviations and names for local service providers and programs if the report is addressed to or might be useful to those unfamiliar with such references. Instead use the local language and then describe the program in general terms. For example, "TSI, a transitional community residential services provider" or "7 West, the alcohol detoxification ward."

Try to be specific about what your statements are based upon. For example, saying that "the client has lost 30 pounds" is probably based on the client's report so don't treat it as a fact or suggest it is based on your own observation unless it is (for example, you might have noted that his clothes seem quite large, a medical history report from a year ago lists a weight 30 pounds greater than you measured, etc).

For the prevention of tampering and loss of pages of a report they can be numbered as "Page 1 of 6", "Page 2 of 6", etc.

# 3.7 Family Genograms:

Enter any relevant information in spaces next to symbols. Use as many copies of the genogram as necessary.

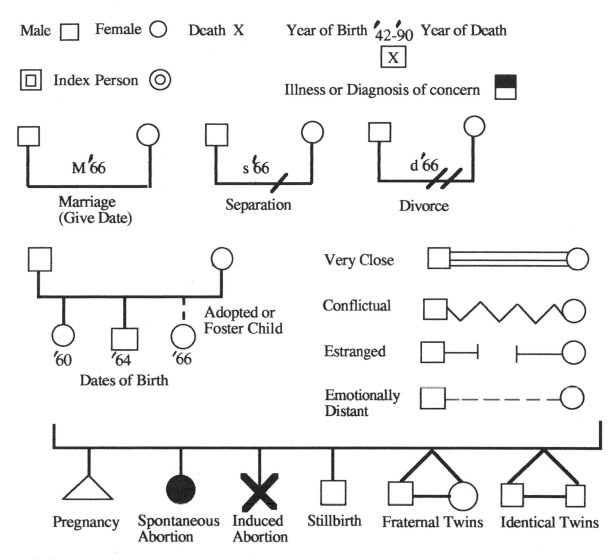

Other symbols:

## 3.8 Abbreviations:

The following are some commonly used and the author's own list of abbreviations found useful:

| | | | | | |
|---|---|---|---|---|---|
| Interview | IV | Intelligence | I | Psychotherapy | P/T |
| Intake | ntk | | | | |
| Psychologist or Psychiatrist | ψ | | | Psychoanalysis | P/A |
| Anyone | AO | No one | NO | Everyone | EO |
| Question | ?, Q | Times (3) | X3 | | |
| Increasing | ↑ | More, greater, larger | > | Present, positive for | ⊕ |
| Decreasing | ↓ | Less, lesser, smaller | < | Not present | ⊖ |
| Occasional | occl | | | | |

| | | | | | |
|---|---|---|---|---|---|
| Summary | Σ | Symptom | Sx | Treatment | Rx or Tx |
| History | Hx | Diagnosis | Dx | Prognosis | Px |
| Homework | HW | History of | h/o | Within normal limits | WNL |
| Discontinued or Discharged | d/c | Status Post | s/p | Prior to Admission | PTA |
| Withdrawal | w/d | After, post | p̄ | Not otherwise specified | NOS |

| | | | | | |
|---|---|---|---|---|---|
| Heart Attack | H/A | Headache | h/a | Diabetes mellitus | DM |
| Depression | D | Anxiety | A | Drug and Alcohol | D+A |
| Paranoia | Pa | Seizures | sz | Mitral Valve Prolapse | MVP |
| Cerebral Vascular Accident | CVA | | | Closed Head Injury | CHI |
| Chronic Obstructive Pulmonary Dis. | COPD | | | Low Back Pain | LBP |
| Motor Vehicle Accident | MVA | | | Hypertension | HBP |

| | | | |
|---|---|---|---|
| Generalized Anxiety Disorder | GAD | Chronic Undifferentiated Schizo. | CUS |
| Delusions and Hallucinations | D+H | Bipolar Affective Disorder | Bip |

| | | | | | |
|---|---|---|---|---|---|
| Date of Birth | DoB | Died | D | Divorced | d |
| Husband | Ⓗ | Daughter | ⓓ | Mother | ⓜ |
| Wife | Ⓦ | Son | Ⓢ | Father | Ⓕ |
| Boyfriend | (bf) | Girlfriend | (gf) | Grandparent | (GP) |
| Sister | Ⓢ | | | | |
| Brother | Ⓑ | Maternal/Paternal Grand Parents | | (MGM)(other) or (MGF)(ather) | |

| | | | | | |
|---|---|---|---|---|---|
| Frequency | f | Number | # | Change | Δ |
| At | @ | Therefore | ∴ | With | c̄ |
| Intercourse | I/C | | | Without | s̄ |

Your own list of preferred abbreviations:

# 4. Mental Status Test Questions/Tasks

## 4.1 Introduction to the Mental Status Questions:

You can, of course, use the questions from the age-appropriate sections of the Binet or the Wechsler subtests of Information, Arithmetic, Comprehension, Similarities or Digit Span for the advantage of precise evaluation of the responses but you may find some of these questions suitable alternatives for subjects who have recently been formally tested or for other reasons.

No assertion or implication of any kind of validity is made nor should be inferred about the use of these questions. As far as I know, there has been no research conducted on them and there are no norms available to guide the clinician in interpreting the responses obtained to the questions asked. The internal "norms" of the experienced and well-trained clinician are the only basis for evaluating such responses.

These areas of mental/cognitive functioning/tasks are LISTED IN ROUGH ORDER OF INCREASING COMPLEXITY and demand on the client because you would probably ask them in this order.

## 4.2 Beginning the Interview:

Always introduce yourself by name and title and obtain fully informed and voluntary consent to the interview (see section 6.8 Informed Consent)

With each client be alert to the client's possible limitations of hearing and vision and inquire if you have any reason to suspect a handicap. Ask for suggestions to improve conditions, such as minimizing the background noise, or changing the lighting. Don't cover your mouth and speak clearly. Take into account the cognitive variations of many of the hearing impaired or users of American Sign Language.

In addition, because of my setting I should remember to always:

Do the following:

Say:

Warn about ...

Explain:

## 4.3 Orientation:

To PERSON: Ask:

"Who are you?"
"What is your name?" (pay attention to nicknames, childhood versions of name, hesitations, aliases)
"Are you married?"
"What kind of work you do/did you do?"

**For a child:** What school do you go to? What grade are you in now?

To PLACE: Ask:

"Where are we/you?" (setting, address/building, city, state/province)
"Where do you live?" (setting, address/building, city, state/province)

To TIME: Ask: (If he/she indicates not knowing ask for a guess or an approximation)

"How old are you?", "When is your birthday?"
"What day is today? Which day of the week is today?, What is today's date?"
"What time is it? Is it day or night?"
"What season is it? What year is it?"
Ask for the dates/duration of hospitalization(s): "When did you first come here?"

To SITUATION: Ask:

"Who am I?"
"What am I doing here?"
"What is the purpose of our talking?"
"Why are you here?"

To FAMILIAR OBJECTS:

Hold up your hand and ask: "Is this my right or left hand?"
                                          "Please name the fingers of my hand."
Hold up/point to a pencil and a watch and ask the S to name the object and its uses

To OTHERS: Ask:

"What is your mother's/father's/spouse's name?"
"What are your children's name(s)?"
"What is my name?"
"What is my title/job?"
"What are the names of some staff members?"  Ask about their titles, functions, etc.
"What are the names of some other patients?"

## 4.4 Attention:
Active information processing about a single or particular stimulus with rejection of distractions or filtering out of irrelevant stimuli. (see section 12.3 Attention)
For Attention Span see sections 4.5 Concentration and 4.8 Immediate memory.


TESTS: (<->) Ask the client to:

"Please say the alphabet as fast as possible." (Note the time taken; normal is 3-10 seconds)
"Spell 'World'/ 'House'. And now, please spell it backward."
"Repeat your Social Security number backwards, please."
*Digit span* forward and reverse. (See section 4.8 Immediate Memory)
Name three objects and have S repeat them or repeat them to the S until all are learned - count the
      trials until the subject is able to repeat accurately.
"Count and then tell me the number of taps I am making." Tap the underside of the table or in some
      other manner make several trials of 3-15 sounds out of the subject's sight.


## 4.5 Concentration:
The maintenance of/holding attention by excluding irrelevant stimuli, or the performance of linked mental acts.

TESTS: (<->)

Ask the subject to "Name the days of the week backwards starting with Sunday."
"Please name the months of the year." "Now please say them backwards."
Ask the subject to "Say the alphabet *backwards* as fast as possible."
"Please tell me as many words as you can think of which begin with the letter F. Don't give me
names/proper nouns or repeat yourself and keep going until I stop you." Stop the subject after
60 seconds and repeat with the letters 'A', 'P', or 'S.' Score is the total number of words meeting
      the criteria on each trial.
Ask the S to write a fairly long and complex sentence from your dictation.
Ask the Subject to tell you when a minute has passed while you talk or don't talk to him/her and record
      the ime taken. Repeat 3 times.
Ask the S to point to/underline each 'A' in a written list presented on a full page of letters: e.g. B,
      F, H, K, A, X, E, P, A, etc.
Mental arithmetic problems: See 4.14 for examples including the famous "Serial Sevens."

## 4.6 Comprehension of Language:

RECEPTIVE: Response to a series of commands such as:

> "Show me how you brush your teeth/comb your hair."
> "Close you eyes, open them, raise an arm, raise your left arm."
> "Put your right hand on your left knee three times and then touch you left ear with your right hand."
> "If today is Tuesday raise one arm, otherwise raise both."
>
> Follows a three stage command - "Pick up that paper, fold it in half, and put it on the floor."
> "Please, read and obey this sentence." (presented on a card): 'Close your eyes.'

EXPRESSIVE:

> Ask him/her to read and explain some sentences from a magazine or newspaper.
> Show him/her a photograph (e.g. in a magazine) and ask for the name(s) of what is depicted.
> Ask him/her to describe a picture portraying several actions.
> "Repeat after me" (one at a time): "One, top, pipe, basket, cabinet, affection, stentorian, pleurisy, Methodist Episcopal; No ifs, ands or buts; liquid linoleum; Third Royal Riding Artillery Brigade."

## 4.7 Eye/hand Coordination/Perceptual-Motor Integration/Dyspraxia/Constructional Ability:

TESTS: Ask the Client to:

> Pick up a coin with each hand.
> Spin a paper clip using each hand.
> Touch each thumb to each finger as you name them (not in order)
> Copy a design of two overlapping pentagons from an illustration on a card.
> Draw a house, a tree, a person, a person of the other sex, themselves.
> Ask the client to draw, from your dictation: a diamond, the outlines of a cross, the edges of a transparent cube, a smoking pipe, a clock face and then indicate the present time as he/she estimates it to be or 'a quarter after six.'

## 4.8 Memory:

**Types:**

*Clinical:* Recognition ("identify, select, pick, or find"), Reproduction ("say, repeat, or copy"), Recall (remember without cueing)
*Theoretical or Processes:* Registration, Retention, Decay, Reproduction
*Kinds:*    Verbal:         words, phrases, stories, associated word pairs
            Visual:         colors, designs, pictures
            Spatial:        positions of objects
            Episodic:       contexts, situations, components, details, sequences, themes
            Practical:      can demonstrate/pantomime how to open a can, brush one's teeth, butter bread

**Tests of Memory:** It is probably best, if it is available, to use the Wechsler *Memory Scale - Revised* or a similar validated test for precise evaluation.

INTRODUCTORY:

> "Has your memory been good?"
> "Have you had any difficulty concentrating or remembering what you read/watch on television/recipes/telephone numbers/appointment times?"
> "Have you recently gotten lost/forgotten an important event/something you were cooking/left some appliance on too long?"
> "Have you had any difficulty recalling people's names or where you know them from?"
> "Have other people suggested to you that your memory is not as good as it was?"

IMMEDIATE memory or memory span (about 10-30 seconds when in the experimental laboratory; what was just said, done or learned during this evaluation when in the clinic):

> *Digit Span*: forward and reverse. "I would like to test your ability to concentrate. I am going to say some numbers one at a time. When I finish please repeat them back to me. Ready?"
> Start with two digits and when repeated correctly on a first or second attempt (with different digits) increase the length of the list by one digit until the Subject fails both trials/number sequences offered. Write the numbers down as you say them, speak at a consistent rate of one digit per second, do not emphasize ending numbers, and avoid consecutive numbers and easily recognizable dates or familiar sequences. Or use you own Social security number or telephone number.
> Then say "Now I am going to say some more numbers but this time I want you to repeat them backward. For example, if I said 6-2, what would you say?"
> The score is the number of correctly recalled digits in correct order. 'Five forward with one mistake' is four forward.
> Normal is about 5-8 forward and 4-6 backward. A difference of 3 or more in maximum Forward minus maximum Backward strongly suggests organically based concentration deficits. Five or more Forward is considered unimpaired in younger or middle-aged adults.

> Ask the subject to "Tap a pencil on the table each and every time I say the letter 'C'". Present a series of random letters at the rate of about 3 each 4 seconds with the letter 'C' randomly distributed but occurring about every 6-8 letters. Normal is making about 1-2 errors (not noticing a 'C') in 30 seconds/45 letters.

## Mental Status Qs

DELAYED RECALL after interference: (variously defined as recall after any intervening activity, few minutes time delay, recent daily events or intra-interview events):

Tell the subject your name and ask him/her to remember it because you will ask for it later. Ask in 5-10 minutes and if not correctly recalled re-inform and teach, then re-ask every 5-10 minutes more and note number of trials to mastery or failure to learn.

Offer 4 items from four categories (E.g. "House, table, pencil, dictionary") and record the number of trials taken to learn the list. Ask for recall in 5-10 minutes. If not recalled prompt with category descriptions (E.g. "A building, a piece of furniture, a writing tool, a kind of book"). If still not recalled ask the subject to select the words from a list of four similar items (E.g. for pencil: pen, crayon, pencil, paintbrush).

Name (for auditory retention) or point to (for visual retention) three items (E.g. Broadway-New York city-taxi; book-pen-tablet; scissors-stapler-pad, apple-peach-pear), tell him or her that you will ask him/her about them later, and then ask him or her to recall them after 5 minutes of interspersed activities.

Give the subject three colors to remember and ask him/her to recall them in 5 minutes.

SHORT-TERM RETENTION: (Short-term retention is a few minutes up to 1-2 hours.)

Have him or her read a narrative paragraph from a magazine or newspaper and produce the gist of the story upon completion without being able to refer to it.

Ask about the events at the beginning of the interview (i.e. Any others present?, What was asked first and next? Which history items were sought).

RECENT memory (a few hours up to 1-4 days, today's events):

Ask about yesterday's meals/television programs/activities/companions (Ask only if these can be verified). Or ask the route taken/distance to this office, the examiner's name (if not over-used in the interview), events in the recent news.

RECENT PAST memory (the last few weeks and months): (Ask only if these can be verified)

"What did you do last weekend?"
"Where did you take your last vacation?"
"What presents did you get on your last birthday/Christmas?"
"What were you doing on the most recent holidays (July 4th, Labor Day, Christmas)?"
"Name any other doctors you have seen, any hospitalizations, tests received, when the present illness began/first felt troubled/ill, etc.?"

REMOTE memory (From approximately 6 months up to all of lifetime or premorbid/symptom onset):

> Client's home address, and phone number.
> "Where were you born?"
> "What is your birth date, your mother's first/maiden name, your first memory?"
> "What was the name of your High School?"
> Ask about childhood events, in correct sequence, places lived, schools attended, names of friends.
> Life history: parents full names, sibling's names and birth order, family deaths, first job, date of marriage, birth dates/ages/names and ages of children.
> Activities on holidays about a year ago or which stand out.
> Local historical events
> Historical events (which you can verify): Sputnik (1957), Watergate (1971), Men landing on the moon (Summer, 1969), name of the President who resigned (Nixon, Aug. 9, 1974), The fall of Saigon (Apr. 29, 1975), Presidents during wars (WW II - Roosevelt, Korean War - Truman, Eisenhower, Viet Nam - Johnson, Nixon), Challenger Disaster (Jan. 28, 1986), etc.

## 4.9 Fund of Information:

BASIC ORIENTATIONS:

> "What is your

| | | | |
|---|---|---|---|
| Birth date? | Social Security number? | Phone number? | Dress size? |
| Address? | Zip code? | Area code? | Waist size? |
| Height? | Weight? | | Shoe size? |

> "Tell me the time." "What time will it be in an hour and a quarter?"
> "How long will it be until Christmas?"
> "How many days are there in a month/year?"
> "Name the days of the week/months of the year."
>
> "Where are we?" (state, county, city, hospital/building, floor, office)
> "Name the local sports teams."
> "What is the capitol of this state?"
> "Which states border this one?"
> "Name five large American cities."
> "How far is it from here to _____ ." (one of the large cities named above).
> "How far is it from New York City to San Francisco?"
> "In which country is Rome/Paris/London/Moscow?"
> "Name three countries in the Middle East/Europe."
> "What is the current population of this city/state/the United States (252 million in 1989), the world (5 billion)?"

# Mental Status Qs

## INFORMATION ABOUT **PEOPLE**:

"Who is the current President? and before him?, and before him? Name the presidents backward starting with the current one." [Presidents of the U.S. since 1900 in reverse order: Bush, Reagan, Carter, Ford, Nixon, Johnson, Kennedy, Eisenhower, Truman, Roosevelt, Hoover, Coolidge, Harding, Wilson, Taft, Roosevelt. Note: The failure to recall these is not diagnostic.]

"Where does the President live?" (in the White House, Washington, D.C.)

"Who was the first President of the United States?"

"Who is the Governor of this state/Mayor of this city?"

"Who is Dr. J., Prince, Michael Jackson, Jesse Jackson, Jackie Robinson, Martin Luther King Jr., Thurgood Marshall, Barbra Jordan?"

"What was George Washington/Thomas Edison/Jonas Salk/Albert Einstein famous for?"

"Who invented the airplane?"

"What does a pharmacist do?"

"Who was JFK?"

## INFORMATION ABOUT **THINGS**:

"Name five foods."

"Name five animals."

"How many sides does a pentagon have?"

"Name three animals beginning with C." [Cat, Cougar, Cow]

"Name three cities beginning with D." [Denver, Detroit, Dallas]

"How many ounces in a pound?"

"What are houses made of?"

"Which is the longest river in the United States?"

"In what direction does the sun rise?"

"Please identify these". (Show some coins and bills of common US currency)

"Who/whose face is on a penny/dollar bill/five dollar bill?"

"At what temperature does water freeze?"

## INFORMATION ABOUT EVENTS:

"What do we celebrate on the 4th of July/Christmas/Thanksgiving Day/Labor Day/Memorial Day/Easter/Passover/Ramadan/Kwansa?"

"Please name some events/big stories that are current/recently in the news/that you have read about in the papers or seen on the TV news."

"What has happened recently in (specify a place)?"

"What did (person's name) do recently? What happened to (person's name) recently?"

"Name some wars the US has been involved in, their dates [World War I (1914-1918) World War II (1939-1945), Korean War/Police action 1950-1953, Viet Nam/Indochina War 1965-1975, Lebanon, Granada, Panama], and the issues involved."

*For those over 50 years of age:*

"What was the date of the attack on Pearl Harbor?" [Dec. 7, 1941]

*For those over 40 years of age:*

"What was the date President John F. Kennedy was assassinated?" [Nov. 22, 1963]

## 4.10 Opposites:

"Please tell me the opposite of each of these words:"

Hard          fast          large          out          high          child

## 4.11 Differences:

Use the format "In what ways are a ____ and a ____ the different or not the same?"

> lie - mistake           duck - robin
> midget - child          orange - baseball
> kite - airplane         water - land

"Which of these is the different one?"
> Desk, <u>apple</u>, chair, lamp. "Why?" [apple in not artificial, not furniture]
> Pottery, statue, painting, poem. "Why?" [<u>Poem</u> is not tactile, <u>Statue</u> does not begin with a 'P']

## 4.12 Similarities:

Use the format "In what ways are a/an _____ and a/an _____ the same or similar?" Question any vague responses until you obtain a clear estimate of the level of comprehension and abstraction involved. For example *train/bus - bicycle* can be interpreted on a spectrum (<->) from "Wheels/people ride on them/means of transportation/technological artifacts."

Ask "Please tell me more about that" and, if necessary, ask "What type/class of things do they belong to?"

EASY:

| | | | |
|---|---|---|---|
| truck/car - bus | duck - chicken | dollar - dime | shoes - pants |
| scissors - saw | book - newspaper | bucket - mug | violin - piano |
| apple - orange | bottle - can | tree - branch | happy - sad |
| car - airplane | ship - airplane | | |

MODERATELY DIFFICULT:

| | | | |
|---|---|---|---|
| door - window | moose - whale | work - play | sun - moon |
| fox - dog | ladder - steps | wings - legs | barn - house |
| cat - lion | bread - milk | tree - forest | |

DIFFICULT:

| | | | |
|---|---|---|---|
| prison - zoo | paper - coal | telephone - radio | theater - church |
| lamp - fan | | | |

## 4.13 Absurdities:

You can, of course, use Absurdities from the Stanford-Binet, Form LM or you might select from your experience examples which are tailored for the particular person being examined. The following are similar to those of the Stanford-Binet, 1980 Revision.

Ask "What is wrong with/foolish/doesn't make sense about this?"

"The doctor rushed into the Emergency Room, got out the bandages, and after eating a sandwich, bandaged the bleeding man."
"Bill's ears were so big he had to pull his sweaters on over his feet."
"An airplane pilot ran out of gas halfway across the ocean so he turned around and flew back to land from where he took off."
"A man was in two auto accidents. The first accident killed him but the second time he got well quickly."

Only if you believe it useful, ask about absurdities/contradictions/paradoxes in everyday life:

The government pays farmers to grow tobacco and also pays for programs to reduce tobacco consumption.
A lemonade mix contains no real lemon but only artificial flavoring and a "lemon" detergent contains real          lemon juice.

## 4.14 Tests of Calculation Abilities:

These require attention, concentration, memory and education. On all math problems make note of the answers given, the effort required/offered, speed and accuracy, changed performance when given a prompt of the next correct answer in a sequence, and/or when given paper and pencil to perform the calculations. Also note self-corrected errors, later self-corrections, use of fingers to count upon, requests for paper and pencil, complaints, excuses, etc.

EXAMPLES: (<->)

"How much is 2+2? And now 4+4? and now 8+8=?" Continue in this sequence and note the limits of skill. More difficult versions are 3+3's and 7+7's.
One-step: $3 + 4 = ?$, $6 \times 4 = ?$,
Two-step: $7 + 5 - 3 = ?$, $8 \times 4 + 9 = ?$, $4 \times 6 \div 3 = ?$

VERBALLY PRESENTED ARITHMETIC PROBLEMS: (<->)

"How many quarters are in $1.75?" [7]
"If oranges are priced at 2 for 18¢, how much would half a dozen cost?" [54¢]
"How much is left when you subtract $5.50 from $14.00?" [$8.50]
"How many nickles are there in one dollar?" [20]
"How many nickles are there in $1.95?" [39]

SERIAL SUBTRACTIONS/ "SERIAL SEVENS":

"Starting with 100 subtract 7 and then subtract 7 from that and continue subtracting 7." Normal is 1 minute or less in subtracting to 2 with 2 or fewer errors (not including spontaneously self-corrections.)

SIMPLER ALTERNATIVES:

Count to 20, count from 1 to 40 by threes, serial 3's subtracted from 31, serial 5's subtracted from 100, serial 4's subtracted from 100

## 4.15 Abstract Reasoning/Proverbs:

Selection of which proverbs to offer depends on your initial assessment of the client' deficits and diagnosis because some are more difficult to interpret satisfactorily while others reveal coping strategies, the intensity of the cognitive dysfunction, or personalization. Say: "What do people mean when they say...?"

PROVERBS WITH THEMES:

All that glitters is not gold; The grass is always greener on the other side; You can't judge a book by its cover (appearances can be deceiving).
Make hay while the sun shines; Strike while the iron is hot (using an opportunity, taking initiative).
Don't cry over spilled/spilt milk (mature resignation and priorities).
Every cloud has a silver lining (depression/pessimism/optimism).
Rome wasn't built in a day; Great oaks from little acorns grow (patience/frustration tolerance/ deferral/delay of gratification).
People who live in glass houses shouldn't throw stones (arrogance, tolerance, guilt, impulse control).
Birds of a feather flock together; Like father like son; The apple doesn't fall far from the tree (the effects of history, genetics or learning).
Don't count your chickens before they are hatched; A bird in the hand is worth two in the bush (caution/realistic hopes/plans).
The squeaking wheel gets the grease (modesty/attention-seeking behavior/self assertion).
A rolling stone gathers no moss (positive and negative interpretations of stones/moss/rolling).
When the cat's away the mice will play (control and rebellion).

Note: It is often advisable to ask if the client has heard these proverbs before.

## 4.16 Paired Proverbs:

These can be used to more carefully evaluate the client's ability, to make subtle distinctions and to hold simultaneously opposing views in mind by presenting them in sequence and without comment.

PROVERBS:

Don't change horses in midstream vs. If at first you don't succeed, try, try again.
A bird in the hand is worth two in the bush vs. Nothing ventured, nothing gained.
Look before you leap vs. He who hesitates is lost/Make hay while the sun shines.
Out of sight, out of mind vs. Distance makes the heart grow fonder.
A stitch in time saves nine vs. Don't cross a bridge until you come to it .
Haste make waste vs. Strike while the iron is hot.

## 4.17 Practical Reasoning:

QUESTIONS:

"Why do we refrigerate many foods?"
"Why do we have newspapers?"
"Why do people buy life/fire insurance?"
"Why should people make a Will?"

HAZARD RECOGNITION: (<->)

"What should you do before crossing the street?"
"Why shouldn't people smoke in bed?"
"What should you do when paper in a wastebasket catches fire?"
"What should you do if grease catches on fire when you are cooking?"

## 4.18 Social Judgement: (see also section 4.17 Practical Reasoning)

QUESTIONS: (<->)

"Why should you go to school?"
"What should you do if you lose a library book?"
"What should you do if you find a purse or wallet in the street?"
"What should you do if you are stopped for speeding?"

"Please tell me of a situation or incident in which you made a foolish or mistaken choice."
"Have you ever been taken advantage of/been a victim?"
"Have you ever made any bad loans?"

"How do you get along with others/people at work?"
"What would you do if someone threatened/tried to hurt you?"
"Please tell me the name of a close friend of yours/someone you would confide in/talk with if you had a personal problem/talk over a serious problem."

"How would you spend $10,000 if it were given to you/you won the lottery?"

"Why do people on an elevator always face the door?"
"What is the role of a free press in a democracy?"
"Why do people feel so strongly about the subject of abortion?"

## 4.19 Self-image:

QUESTIONS:

"Please describe your personality."
"How would you describe yourself?"
"Which three words best describe you?"
"If you could be any animal, which would you choose and why?"
"Would/could/can you identify the turning points in your life?"
"What would be written on your tombstone/in your obituary if you were to die today?"
"Has life been fair to you?"

## 4.20 Insight: (for descriptors of responses see section 13.12 Insight)

GENERAL:

"Why are you here?", "What causes you to be here?"
"What kind of place is this? What goes on here?"
"Why are you seeing me?"
"What do you think has caused your troubles/being disabled/being hospitalized?"
"What changes would help you most?"

INTO ILLNESS:

"Do you think there is something wrong with you? What? Do you think you are ill?"
"Did you ever have a nervous breakdown/bad nerves/something wrong with your mind?"
"Do you think you need treatment?"
"Why did/do you need to take medicines?"
"Did you come here voluntarily?"
"What are your suggestions for your treatment?"

## 4.21 Background Information Related to Mental Status:(See also section 7 Background Information)

"How far did you go in school/how many grades did you finish in school/did you finish High
School?"
"In school were you ever left behind a grade/not promoted to the next grade/ have to take a grade
over again?"
"Were you ever in any kind of special classes/special education/classes for the learning
disabled/slow learners/retarded/socially and emotionally disturbed or disabled?"

**Mental Status Qs**

Notes and Additions/Suggestions:

# 5. Inquiries for Signs, Symptoms and Syndromes of Disorders

This list of questions excludes all those topics referring to Cognitive or Mental Status functioning (which are covered in section 4. Mental Status Examination Questions). Topics here are in alphabetical order as no hierarchy is agreed upon.

## Abuse

Alcohol/Drug: (see section 5.23 Substance abuse)

## 5.1 Physical/Spouse:

Inquire of all patients about physical abuse, threats, fights, arguments

## 5.2 Abused Child:

PHYSICAL ABUSE (Note: Obtain medical consultation if you have suspicions about injuries)

Look for evidence of injuries and inquire how they occurred and what was done about them. Attend to:

Explanations of the cause of the injury and especially any reluctance to explain, and different explanations by different care-givers
Whether treatment was sought in a timely and effective fashion
Previous similar or suspicious injuries
Cooperation with previous treatments prescribed
Risk factors: unwanted birth, prematurity, poverty, developmental delay, "difficult baby", colicky baby, inappropriate expectation, poor baby/parent match, many small children, few supports, previous involvement with the authorities, drug or alcohol abuse, etc.
Psychological patterns such as depression, anxiety, avoidance, preference for isolation, acting out, etc.

If the injury was the result of disciplining the child inquire about when they discipline and how and what so annoyed the care-giver as to result in the injury

SEXUAL ABUSE (Note: This is a speciality area; if you are not experienced and trained get consultation or refer before going very far into the topic for fear of contaminating the truth)

"What do you call your private parts? What do you call the other sex's private parts?"

"Who has touched your private parts?" (Note: Do not add "when you didn't want them to" as that may not have been true or is yet unrecognized.)
"Who, when, where, why?"
"Whom did you tell? What did they do about it?"

## 5.3 Affect/Mood: (See also sections 5.4 Anxiety and 5.10 Depression)

"How would you describe your mood today?"
"Are you happy, sad or what right now?"
"When are/were you happiest?"
"Using a scale where plus 10 is as happy as you have ever been, 1 is not depressed at all and minus
　　10 is as depressed as you have ever been, please rate your mood today."
"What is your usual mood like?"  If negative ask "When was it last good?"
"What was your mood like during your childhood/adolescence/earlier life?"
"Were there ever times when you couldn't control your feelings?"

## 5.4 Anxiety:

"How does the future look to you?"
"What do you worry about?"
"Is there something you are very concerned about/afraid of happening?"

"When you get frightened what happens to you?"
"Do you ever have times of great fear or anxiety/panic attacks?" (Inquire about cues/triggers,
　　frequency, duration, whether observed by others, specific physiological symptoms, the
　　sequence of the symptoms, etc.)

"Are there any distressing memories which keep coming back to you?"

"Is there any situation you avoid because it really upsets/scares you?"

## 5.5 Chronic Pain:

"Do you frequently have pain somewhere in your body? Where?"
"Does the pain keep you from doing the things you want to/working/interfere with your sex life/in
　　some other way or ways limit you?"
"Do you have to lie down and rest because of the pain or does it force you to keep moving?"
"Do you find that you are thinking about the pain a lot?"

"Which medicines do you usually take for the pain?"
"Do doctors seem to have failed you?"
"Has some doctor said your pain was 'imaginary' or 'all in your head'?"
"Do you secretly think you case is hopeless?"

## 5.6 Compliance/Non-Compliance:

"What problems have you had in getting treatment/finding an understanding doctor/keeping scheduled medical appointments?"
"What problems have you had in taking prescribed medications?"
"What medications are you taking?" "What medications should you be taking?"
"Have you ever stopped taking the medications prescribed before they ran out/because of some reason?" "What was the reason?"
"Is there anything which makes you reluctant to take medications prescribed for you?"

## 5.7 Compulsions: (see also section 5.16 Obsessions)

"Are you a person who is especially careful about safety?"
"Is there anything in your house/at work that you have to check on frequently?"
"Do you have to check the doors/windows/locks/kitchen/house/your family's safety?"

"Do these actions seem reasonable to you?"
"Do you feel uncomfortable until these actions are done, even though you may know them to be unimportant/even foolish/that they won't really work?"

"Do you have any habits/frequent actions/rituals/behaviors that you must/feel compelled to do in a particular way or very often?"
"Is there some things you must do in order to fall asleep?"
"Are there any actions you have to do before or while you eat/go to the bathroom?"
"Do you ever have to arrange your clothes in certain ways?"
"Are you very careful about /afraid of poisons/dirt/germs/diseases/contamination?"

"Are there any words or phrases you feel that you have to say in a certain way or at certain times?"

## 5.8 Delusions: False (unaccepted by society/subculture/peers), fixed/change-resistant beliefs. (see also section 5.18 Paranoia)

CONTROL:

"Did anyone try to read your mind/use unusual means to force thoughts into your mind/try to take/block some of your thoughts away/stop or block your thoughts?"
"Did you ever hear a voice telling you what to do?"
"Have you ever been forewarned/known that something would happen before it did?"

GRANDEUR/SPECIAL ABILITIES:

> "Are you an especially gifted person?" [Note reports of a large number of cars or other possessions, exaggerated abilities, titles/degrees/education/high positions/dramatic or unlikely consumption of alcohol or drugs or history of unlikely or criminal activities]
> "Do you have great wealth/unusual strengths/special powers/impressive sexual potency?"
> "Are you able to influence others/read people's minds/put thoughts in their minds?"
> "Do/did you ever receive personal messages from heaven/God/someone unusual?"
> "Have you been in communication with aliens/dead people/God/Christ/the Devil/the Blessed Virgin/any Biblical persons?"
> "Do you think you are immortal/cannot be harmed/hurt/killed?"

IMPOSTER:

> "Are you a fake?" [Separate a delusion from beliefs of inadequacy based on low self-esteem]
> "Do you think people recognize who you really are?"
> "Are you concerned about being discovered/identified/exposed?"
> "What is your real rank?"

MONOMANICAL:

> Is this person preoccupied with a certain ideas, themes, events or persons? Does all his/her conversation return to a single topic/false idea?

NIHILISTIC:

> "Do you think everything is lost/hopeless?"
> "Do you think that tomorrow will never come?"
> "Do you think that the world has stopped?"
> "Do you think that things outside no longer exist?"
> "Do you still have all the parts of your body?"

PERSECUTION: (see section 5.18 Paranoia)

REFERENCE:

> "Do people do things/do things happen which only you really understand/have special meanings for you/are designed to convey or tell you something no one else is to know?"
> "Are things you see on the radio/TV or read in the papers especially meaningful to you/contain special messages just for you?"

SOMATIC/HYPOCHONDRIACAL:

"How is your health? How often are you ill? How often do you see a physician? Do you have many illnesses/medical or health problems?"

"Do you have a lot of pain or unusual pains?"

"Which medicines do you take regularly? Which medicines do you take regularly that don't need a prescription?"

"Is there some illness you are worried about getting or that you already have that worries you?"

"How often do you think about it?"

"How does it make you feel when you think about it?"

"What do you do about it?"

"Do you think you might/have a serious disease like cancer or AIDS or MS?"

"Do you think you might/have some horrible disease which hasn't been diagnosed correctly or has no cure?"

"Do you think you have a serious disease but haven't been able to find a doctor to treat it?"

SELF-DEPRECIATION: (see also section 5.10 Depression)

"Do you think you are worthless/sinful/ugly/emitting bad/noxious odors/will be punished because you have sinned unforgivably?"

## 5.9 Depersonalization and Derealization:

DEPERSONALIZATION:

"Are you aware of any significant change in yourself?"

"Do you feel normal/alright/natural/real?"

"Do you ever feel that you have lost your identity/like you were someone else?"

"Are you always certain who you are?"

"Do you ever wonder who you really are?"

"Did you ever feel that you were no longer real/you were becoming someone or something different?"

"Did you ever feel that your self/body was different/changed/unreal/strange?"

"Ever feel like you were/your mind was outside/watching/apart from yourself/your body?"

"Have there been times you felt your mind and body were not together/linked?"

"Do you ever feel like someone else was moving your legs as you walked/ever felt like a robot?"

DEREALIZATION:

"Did you ever feel like you weren't really present?"

"Ever feel you were detached/alienated/estranged from yourself or your surroundings/everything around you?"

"Did you ever feel that things around you/the world were/was very strange/remote/unreal/changing?"

"Do things seem natural and real to you?"

"Do people, trees, houses, etc. look as they usually do/always did to you?"

"Did things or objects ever seem to be alive?"

"Ever get so involved in a daydream that you couldn't tell if it were real or not?"

## 5.10 Depression:

SOMATIC/VEGETATIVE SYMPTOMS:

"How is your general health? Has it changed recently?" [Follow up reports of symptoms]
"Has your interest in food increased or decreased?"
"Have you gained or lost weight?"
"How is your sleep? Do you have trouble falling asleep? On how many nights in a week?"
"Do you wake in the middle of the night, other than to go to the bathroom, and then can't get back to sleep?"
"Do you wake early and can not fall asleep again?"
"Do you regularly nap during the day?" [Count this into total sleep hours which decrease with age]
"Have your bowel or bladder habits changed?"
"Has your interest in sex changed?" [Libido is desire not performance]

AFFECTIVE SYMPTOMS:

"How are your spirits generally?"
"How did you feel about (specific event/life in general)?"
"When was the last time you felt really down?" Do you get pretty discouraged/depressed/blue? Are you blue/feeling low now? Do you get sad or down for long?
"Have you felt some personal losses recently?"
"Do you think you are more depressed in the winter than the summer or only in one season?"
        [Consider Seasonal Affective Disorder]
"Have you had a time when you felt very tired or very irritable?"

SOCIAL FUNCTIONING:

"Have you given up friendships?"
"Do you find yourself avoiding people?"

SUICIDAL IDEATION:

"When people are depressed they sometimes think about dying. Have you had thoughts like that?"
"Are there times when you wish you would not wake up?"
"Do you feel that life isn't worth living? Do you think you would just as soon be dead/that things/other people would be better off if you were dead?"
"Have you been troubled by thoughts of hurting yourself?, When was the last time you thought of doing away with/killing yourself?" (see 5.25 Suicide)


"Do you think you will get well/over this problem? How?"
"What do you see for yourself in the future?"

"What is the worst thing that ever happened to you?"
"What is the best thing that ever happened to you?"
"If you could have three wishes come true, what would you wish for?"

SELF-DEPRECATION:

"Are you hard on yourself?"
"Do you think you are a wicked person?, Why? Do you think that you have sinned and cannot be forgiven?"

**Drug Abuse** (see section 5.23 Substance Abuse)

ALWAYS ask every client about use and history of medications/street drugs/alcohol/other chemicals

## 5.11 Eating Disorders:

"Have you gained or lost weight in the last year? How much?"
"How often do you think about your weight or eating?"
"How do you feel about your current weight?" [Note any disparity between client's statements and appearance]
"Do you feel you are (always) too fat?", "Are you afraid of being or becoming overweight?"
"How would your life be different if you lost the weight you want to?"

"What kinds of diets have you tried?" [Take a diet history]
"Have you ever gotten so upset or desperate about your weight that you have done something drastic?"
"Have you ever: gone on eating binges, vomited after you've eaten, fasted for long periods, used diet pills/cathartics/laxatives/diuretics to lose weight, lost a great deal of weight, or felt guilty after eating?"

See also Garner and Garfinkel (1979) for anorexia nervosa.

## 5.12 Hallucinations: sensory perceptions independent of consensual reality/stimuli noticeable by others.
If there is an indication of the presence of hallucinations ask questions to eliminate those apparently due to entering or leaving sleep, delirium, alcohol or drug withdrawal or abuse.

GENERAL QUESTIONS:

"Do you have a vivid imagination?"
"Do you dream vividly/so you aren't sure it was a dream?"
"Did you ever think/act in really strange/odd/peculiar ways?"
"Did you ever see or hear things others did not?"
"Have you had any uncanny experiences/anything ever happened to you you cannot explain?"

AUDITORY:

"Have you ever heard noises in your head that disturb you?"
"Have you ever heard voices or sounds that other people didn't hear/someone calling your name or talking to you when no one was there?"
"Have you ever heard voices coming from inside your head?"
"Was this your own thoughts as if a voice were speaking to you or some other voice?"
 Where do the voices come from?"
"Whose voice?, Man's or women's?, How old were they?, What did they say?, When does this happen?, How often do you hear them?, What brings these on?"

YVONNE DAVIS

## Sx Qs

VISUAL:

"Have you ever seen anything so unusual that other people didn't believe it?"
"Did you ever have visions/apparitions/ghosts?"
"Did you ever see anything like in a dream when you were awake?"
"Have you ever seen things that no one else saw?, What?, What did you feel then?, What do you call these experiences?, What causes these things to happen?"

KINESTHETIC:

"Have you ever felt strange sensations/odd feelings in your body/anything crawling on you?"

GUSTATORY:

"Have you ever felt strange tastes in your mouth?" (poison in your food, metal, electricity, etc.)

OLFACTORY:

"Have you ever smelled strange odors which you could not account for?" (poisons, death, something burning, sewage, odd smells from your own body, dead spirits, etc.)

OTHER:

"What was the strangest experience you ever had?, Did you ever visit another planet?, Ever die and return to life?"
"How do you think these things come about?

Note: If Subject denies hallucinations note these behaviors which suggest hallucinating: return of gaze to a spot, sudden head turning, staring at one place in room, eyes following something in motion, mumbling or conversing with anyone else, etc.

---

## 5.13 Illusions: misinterpretations or misperceptions of sensory stimuli. (see also section 5.9 Derealization)

"Do things ever seem to change size/look smaller, or larger?"
"Do parts of your body ever seem to change in size or shape or texture?"
"Do things sometimes seem nearer or farther away that they should?"
"Does the world look very different to you?" "In what way(s)?"
"Do any things feel different, in some way, at certain times?"
"Does time ever seem to move very slowly or very fast/telescope?"
"Were you ever surprised that you could hear some sounds other people couldn't hear?" (e.g. whispering voices, echoes, very loud common sounds, etc.)

## 5.14 Impulse Control:

"Do you find yourself suddenly doing things before you have thought about or decided to do them?"
"Do you feel compelled/driven to do things you don't want to do?"
"Do you feel unable to stop yourself from doing some things?"

"Have you ever been involved in sexual behaviors you regretted?"
"Ever steal/shoplift?
"Please tell me about all the times you have had contact with the police."
"Do you get involved in more fights than others in your neighborhood?"
"Have you ever been fired/evicted/arrested? Why did that happen?"

"What do you usually do when you get very upset and angry?"
"Do you have a bad temper/fly off the handle/flare up?"
"Have you ever lost control of yourself? Ever thrown/broken things? Ever hit/attacked anyone?"

## Insight: (see sections 4.20 Insight questions and 13.12 Insight descriptors)

## 5.15 Mania: (see also section 10.6 Mania)

"Was there ever a time when you were very excited/talked too much/been restless/did without sleep without having any reason?"
"Were you ever too happy/full of energy/oversexed/spent money recklessly/started things you couldn't finish?"
"Was there ever a time when you were too impatient/irritable/couldn't concentrate?"
"When did this start? How long did this last? What happened because of this? Were you ever treated for this condition?"

## 5.16 Obsessions: (see also section 5.7 Compulsions, and 12.7 Preoccupations)

"Are there any thoughts you just seem not to be able to forget/get rid of/keep out of your mind/stop thinking about?"
"Is there anything your thoughts revolve around or continually come back to?"
"Are there any phrases/names/dates/slogans/rhymes/titles/music that continually run through your mind/you can't seem to control?"
"Are there any prayers/numbers/names/phrases you feel you have to repeat? When?"

"Is there any possibility you keep thinking about/considering/mulling over/speculating about?"
"Are there any everyday decisions you seem unable to make or spend an excessive length of time making?"
"How often do you think about your health or how your body is working or if it is sick?"

## 5.17 Organicity:

Ask for a HISTORY of:

| | | |
|---|---|---|
| Sunstroke | Head injuries | Periods of unconsciousness/knocked out/having |
| Near-drowning | Head surgery | fainted |
| Electrocution | Apnea | High fevers/delirium |
| Poisonings | Vertigo/dizziness | Seizures/convulsions/fits |

Exposure to toxic chemicals in the workplace
Substance use/abuse/overdoses (see section 5.23 Substance abuse)

Consider neuropsychological testing and/or neurological evaluations.

## 5.18 Paranoia:

BEING MONITORED:

"When you get on a bus or enter a restaurant do people notice you/turn around to look at you?"
"Are people talking about you? Do people say things about you behind your back? What do they say?"
"Have you ever been watched/spied on/singled out for special attention?"
"Do people sometimes follow you for a while?"

SUSPICION:

"Are you very concerned about what others think about you?"
"Did people laugh at you/talk about you behind your back?"
"Are people are making insulting/derogatory/critical/negative remarks about you?
"Did people ever think you were homosexual when you weren't?"

"Do you think anyone is against you?"
"Do you believe you have to be extra careful/extra alert/vigilant around people?"
"Are people doing things which affect you and which you do not understand?"
"Would you say that you are more suspicious than other people, perhaps with good cause?"

PLOTTED AGAINST:

"Do you think there is someone or something out to get you?"
"Do you have enemies?"
"Is there anything about you which has made other people prejudiced against/out to get/harm you or damage your property?"
"Does any organization or group of people have it in for you/plotting against you?"
"Have you been attacked/been shot at? Do you need to carry a gun/knife/Mace/hire a body-guard?"

BEING CONTROLLED:

"Do people try to trick you/play tricks on you?"
"Do other people seem to know your thoughts? Can other people read your mind?"
"Have you ever had thoughts in your mind which were not your own?"
"Are people controlling your thoughts or your mind? What are they doing? How are they attempting this?, Why is this happening?"
"Is your mind controlled by other's/thought waves/electricity/radio or television waves?"
"Are there drugs in your food or drinks?"

## 5.19 Phobias:

"Are you afraid of any things that do not frighten most people as much? What are they?"
"Is there anything or any place(s) that make(s) you very uncomfortable or anxious and so you avoid it/them?"
"Are there any places/things/activities you must avoid? Why?"
"Do these fears/behaviors seem reasonable to you?"
"What have you tried to overcome these fears?"

## 5.20 Sexual History: (This section is for a non-problem focussed history, see sections 7.6 for Sexual Adjustment, and 10.7 for Attitudes and Behaviors. See Pomeroy, et al.. (1982) for how to take a very complete sexual history)

ALWAYS ask every client about a history of sexual abuse. (See section 5.1 Sexual Abuse Questions)

CHILDHOOD:

"When were you first aware of the sexes' differences?"
"What sex games did you play with girls and with boys?"
"Did anyone ever touch you sexually when you didn't want them to?" (See section 5.1 Sexual Abuse)
"What were your first sexual feelings? How old were you? What was the situation? What thoughts did you have then?"
"When you saw someone involved in sexual activity what was your reaction?"

ADOLESCENCE:

"Did you feel free to ask sexual questions in your home?" "To whom/where did you go with your questions/for information?"
"When did you first masturbate? How did you learn about masturbation? What did it feel like and what did you think when you started?"
"How and when did you learn about menstruation and pregnancy?"
"How prepared were you for menstruation/wet dreams/the changes in your body?"
"What was you first experience with petting like? With intercourse? Homosexual experience?
"At what age did you start to date?"
"How old were you when you first had sex with another prson?"
    "Was this heterosexual or homosexual?"
Questions for females: age of menarche, ir/regularities of menstrual cycle, changes in menstrual cycle, pregnancies/miscarriages/abortions/deliveries
Questions for males: age of puberty (voice cracking, nocturnal emissions, body hair, orgasm by masturbation, etc.)

ADULTHOOD:

"How many sexual partners have you had? How many have been pick-ups/one-night-stands, prostitutes, married persons?

"Which sexually transmitted diseases have you had?

"Have you had sexual experiences with people of you own sex?

"Who, if anyone, have you had a sexual experience with who was also a relative of yours?

"Have you ever forced anyone to have sex with you? Have you ever been forced to have sex with anyone?"

"What are your sexual fantasies about? Do any of your sexual fantasies distress or frighten you?"

"Do you have any sexual problems now? Did you in the past? Which?"

    For Men:

        "When have you had difficulty with erection/orgasm/ejaculation?

    For Women:

        "When have you had difficulty with arousal, or orgasm?"

"As you see it, do these affect you alone, mainly you, you and your partner, or is it mainly your partner's problem?"

"What have you done to try to overcome this/these problem?"

[Ask about use of medications - prescription and over-the-counter, street drugs, alcohol (by referring to sections 5.23 and 5.24) and about intercurrent illnesses especially diabetes]

    For Women:

        "How does your menstrual cycle affect your mood/attitudes/behavior/sexual desire?"

        "Please describe all your pregnancies."

RELATIONSHIPS:

"If you have been married before, what was the nature of the sexual relationship? What was the reason the relationship ended?"

"In your present relationship, how has the sexual adjustment been?"

"How attracted to your partner do you feel?"

"How attractive do you feel to your partner?"

"Are you satisfied with the frequency of sexual relations? Is your partner?"

"What images or fantasies do you think of when you are with your partner?"

"What conflicts do you have with your partner in any aspect of your sexual relationship?" (oral sex, positions, frequency, amount of stimulation, the circumstances of sex, communication of preferences, initiation, etc.)

"What incompatibilities or conflicts exist in other aspects of the relationship?"

## 5.21 Sexual Identity:Transsexuality [Distinguish transexuality from transvestism, cross dressing, dissatisfaction with one's body and delusions]

"At what age did you first know you were a boy/girl?"
"Did you ever dress in the other sex's clothes/play with their toys?"
"Do you want to look like someone of the other sex?"
"Do you think you really should have been/are the other sex?"
"Are your sex organs normal? Do you dislike them?"
"Do you dislike your sex's clothes or bodies?"
"Have you ever sought to change your sex?"
"Do you want to marry a person of your sex?"

FOR FEMALES:

"Were you a tomboy? Are you still?"
"Do you stand up to urinate?"
"Do you feel like a man trapped in a woman's body?"

FOR MALES:

"Do you ever dress in women's clothes?, makeup?, underclothes only?"
"When do you do this? How does it make you feel? What do you get from this?"
"Do you feel like a woman trapped in a man's body?"

## 5.22 Sleep:

GENERAL QUESTIONS:

"Do you have any trouble with your sleep? What kind?"
"How much sleep do you usually get each night?"
"Do you wake up refreshed?"
"What time do you usually go to bed? fall asleep? wake up, get up?" [Note total sleep time for age and
        lifelong normality]
"Has there been any change in the ways you sleep?"
"Are you sleepy during the day? Do you usually/have to take a nap during the day?"
"Do you snore loudly?"
"What do you dream about? Do you have bad or unusual dreams?"
"Do you have nightmares/frightening dreams?
"Do you usually have the same dream every night for a while?"
"Are there dreams you dream over and over?"

DIFFICULTY FALLING ASLEEP

"Typically, what time do you go to bed?"
"Typically, what time do you fall asleep?"
"Does it take you more than 20 minutes to fall asleep after you go to bed?"
"What keeps you awake? (activities, partner, rehearsing the day, conditions of bedroom) What do you
        think about before you fall asleep?"
"Do you see or hear or feel unusual things before falling asleep?"
"What do you do in bed?" (watch TV, read, study, use telephone. have sex, etc.)
"Do you do anything to help yourself fall asleep? What do you do to fall asleep?"

SLEEP CONTINUITY DISTURBANCE:

"How well do you sleep? Are you a very/light/sound/very sound sleeper?"
"Do you awaken in the middle of the night? What awakens you?"
"Is there anything which wakes you so you can't sleep through the night? (need to urinate, your bed
        partner's behavior, a needy child, street noises, etc.)
"Are you able to return to sleep in 15 minutes or less? If not how long do you stay awake?"
"What do you think about as you lie in bed? What have you tried to return to sleep?"

EARLY MORNING AWAKENING:

"What time do you usually wake up/awaken?"
"Do you awaken early in the morning and are unable to go back to sleep again?"
"What do you think about as you lie in bed?"

OTHER:

"How much coffee/cola/tea do you drink each day?, Do you use any caffeine containing medications
        such as Midol, Bufferin, Anacin, etc.?"
"How many cigarettes do you smoke in a day?"
"Do you awaken gasping for air/with leg jerks or cramps or pain?"
"What medications are you taking?"
"What do you eat before going to sleep?"
"Do you work shiftwork/changing/rotating shifts?"

## 5.23 Substance Abuse/Drugs and Alcohol:

Note: At present, substance abuse and misuse issues concern:
> Alcohol
> Prescription/legal drugs such as amphetamines, barbiturates, inhalants, opiods, sedatives, hypnotics, and anxiolytics
> Street/illegal/unidentified/designer drugs such as cannabis, cocaine, hallucinogens
> Over-the-counter medications
> Caffeine containing beverages and foods,
> Tobacco

There are no sharp demarcations or agreed upon criteria between use, misuse, abuse, being an 'alcoholic', 'problem drinker', or 'alcohol addict'.

DSM III-R criteria for dependence: At least 3 of the following items: 1) use of greater than intended amounts or use of over a longer than intended period, 2) unsuccessful attempts to reduce or control use, 3) extensive time spent in obtaining, using or recovering from use of the substance, 4) being intoxicated or withdrawing when expected to fulfil role obligations, or when use is physically dangerous, 5) abandonment or reduction of significant social, occupational or recreational activities because of use, 6) use despite knowing of its causing or worsening a social, psychological or physical problem, 7) **tolerance** so one needs ∫more for intoxication, and, for some substances, 8) characteristic **withdrawal** symptoms, and lastly, 9) use of the substance to control or avoid withdrawal symptoms. Ratings of severtiy are made for dependence: mild, moderate, severe, in partial or full remission

Note: Because the individual's patterns of use/overuse/misuse/abuse change with availability, resources, setting, choice, treatment and aging, and may involve cross-addictions, temporary substitutions or preferences a detailed and individualized history is desirable. However, such tailoring is not possible in the format here. Therefore follow the client's lead in history taking to get all the relevant facts and experiences.

GENERAL QUESTIONS ABOUT EFFECTS:

"What is/are your drugs of choice/preference?"
"What problems has the use of alcohol/drugs caused in your life at any time? Has drinking/drug use caused you any problems in the last month?"
"Has drinking/drug use affected your school/work/job/career, friendships/family/marriage, health, or any other area of your life?"
"What happens to you when you drink/use drugs? Do you change a lot/act very differently/do strange things/have other parts of your personality come out?"
"When did you lose control over your drinking/drug use?"
"Are you or other people concerned about your drinking/drug use? Have people tried to get you to stop drinking/using?"
"What is the longest period in your life in which you didn't drink or use drugs?"

CONSUMPTION PATTERNS:

## Alcohol:

"When and where did you first drink any kind of alcohol?"
"When and where did you first drink to excess/drunkenness?"
"When did you first start drinking regularly?"
"Do you drink more now?"
"How did you progress to the quantity you now drink?"

"What is your preferred drink?"
"Do you ever drink alcohol substitutes such as shaving lotion or hair tonic?"
"Do you drink every day or every other day?"
"When you drink how much do you consume? Do you drink a case of beer/fifth of whiskey in a day/drink for two days in a row?"
"At what time of day do you start drinking?" "When do you drink?" (as soon as awaken/all day long/no particular time/at lunch/after work/with dinner/late at night/weekends only)
"Do you ever feel you *need* a drink to get going/can't get through the day without a drink?"

"What are the usual situations or moods just before you start drinking?"
"Do you ever drink heavily after a fight or disappointment?"
"Do you drink more when you feel under a great deal of pressure?"

"Where do you get your alcohol?" (from peers/dealers/bartenders/steal it/sneak it from others)
"Where do you drink?" (at work/home/parties/bars)
"With whom do you drink?" (alone/with buddies/friends/spouse)
"Do you drink now without eating anything?"
"When you are drinking at a party or social occasion do you sneak a few extra drinks?"
"Do you gulp your drinks to get drunk quickly?"
"Do you conceal/lie about the amount of your drinking?"

## Drugs:

"What drugs have you used?" (street drugs like marijuana/cocaine/crack/heroin/ice/hallucinogens/ LSD/"Ecstasy"/"uppers"/"speed"/"downers"/pain killers/"ludes"/"Reds"/"Black Beauties"/ tranquilizers/etc.?)
"What chemicals have you used?" (glue sniffing, inhalants such as gasoline, butane, naptha, etc.)
"What drugs or medications have you used in the last month/6 months? How did you get them?"
"Have you ever used drugs prescribed for you (such as pain killers/sleeping pills/tranquilizers/ barbiturates/etc.) in a way that the doctor didn't prescribe?"
"Have you ever taken medications prescribed for someone else?"

"When did you first use street drugs or misuse medications or sniff chemicals?"
"What effects did they have on you?"
"What did you use at first?"
"When did you first start using it/them regularly?"
"How did you progress to the quantity you now use?"

"What are the usual situations or moods just before you start using?"
"How often do you use? When do you start using? Do you ever feel you *need* to do some drug just to get going/get through the day or night?"
"Where do you use?" (at work/home/parties/houses)
"With whom do you use?" (alone/with buddies/friends/spouse)
"How do you take each drug/chemical? What is the usual/maximum amount you take?"

*The following sets of questions apply to both alcohol and drugs:*

CONTROL:

"When was the first time you became concerned about your use of drugs or alcohol?"
"Have you failed to keep promises to yourself to cut down on your drinking/drugs?"
"Why do you stop? What stops you?" (Internal or external forces)
"Have you ever tried to cut down or stop and couldn't? What thoughts/feelings/urges did you have when you tried to stop or refrain?"
"What means have you tried to control your drinking/drug use?" (relocating, prayer/religion, switching to (beer), willpower, detoxification, rehabilitation programs, Alcoholics Anonymous, etc.)
"What was the longest period of sobriety/staying clean you have had?"
"Do you ever lie about/conceal/justify/avoid discussion of your actual drinking/drug use?"
"What are the positive and negative effects of your drinking/drug use? What are the effects you like best?
"Have you ever regretted what you have done or said when you were drunk/high?"

HEALTH CONSEQUENCES:

"Did a doctor ever tell you to stop drinking/using drugs for your health?"
"Have you ever received treatment/medication/been in a hospital because of your drug use/drinking/drinking too much/for detoxification from drinking/drug use?"

"Have you ever had any of these when you drank or stopped drinking: shakes/morning tremors, visions, hearing voices, feeling things on your skin, D.T.'s (Delirium Tremens), cirrhosis, gastritis, pancreatitis, convulsions, jaundice, or any other disease or problem?"
"Have you ever had blackouts/times where you couldn't remember what you did or how you got to where you were? When did these first happen and when most recently? How often?"
"Have you ever become very drunk when you had only one or two drinks?"

FAMILY CONSEQUENCES/IMPACTS:

"Have your friends/family members complained/showed concern about your drinking/drug use?"
"Have you ever gotten into a serious fight with/hit/beaten/been beaten by your spouse/children when drunk/high?"
"Is your partner also a problem drinker/alcoholic/drug abuser?"
"Do any family members like your brothers or sisters/parents/children have a problem with alcohol or drugs?"
"Does or did chemicals cause strained relations with you children or family/neglect/verbal/sexual/ physical abuse?"
"Is there a history of physical/sexual/emotional abuse in your family or the family you came from?"
"Does drinking ever spoil family gatherings/make for a atmosphere of tension/make your children afraid of you/cause others to talk about you?"
"Do you avoid your family when you are drinking/high?"
"Has drinking/drug use caused you any sexual problems?"
"How would you describe the overall effect of drinking/drugs on your marriage/children/family/ friends?"
"Do you feel guilty/embarrassed/remorseful/apologetic about the way you drink/use drugs?"

VOCATIONAL/FINANCIAL CONSEQUENCES:

"Did your drinking/drug use ever cause problems when you were in school?"
"How much work have you missed because you were drunk/high/hung over?"
"Did you ever get into fights at work?"
"If you were in the military did you drink there? Did your drinking cause problems in the military?"
"Have you ever been disciplined/fired/damaged anything/hurt anyone because of your drinking/drug
       use?"

"How did/do you get the money to buy drugs?"
"How much dealing in drugs have you done?"

LEGAL CONSEQUENCES:

"Have you been arrested for being drunk/disorderly conduct, Driving While Intoxicated/Driving
       Under the Influence, assault or other crimes/destructive behavior when you were drunk?"
"Have you gotten into fights while you were drunk/high?"
"Have you run up large debts/been evicted because of drinking or drug use?"

OTHER ASPECTS:

"What kind of person are you when you are drunk/high?"
"Has your drinking/drug use caused you any spiritual problems?"
"Would you say you are a "social drinker" or "have a drinking problem" or how would you describe
       your use?"
"Do you think you are addicted?" "Do you think you are an alcoholic?"

---

## 5.24 Substance Use - Cigarettes and Caffeine

TOBACCO

"Do you smoke cigarettes/cigars/a pipe?"
"Do you chew/use smokeless tobacco/snuff?"
"How many cigarettes/cigars do you smoke each day?"
"When did you start smoking?"
"Did you ever smoke more or less than you do now?"
"Have you changed the brand you smoke to cut down?"
"Have you tried to stop smoking? How? How many times? What has and hasn't worked for you?"

CAFFEINE:

"How many cups of coffee (except decaffeinated/Sanka) or cola drinks (Coke, Pepsi, Dr. Pepper, etc.
       diet or regular) do you drink in a day?" [Note: some non-cola drinks contain caffeine]
"How often do you take APCs/Anacin/Bufferin/(for pre-menopausal females) Midol?"
"How often do you eat chocolate?" "Do you have some chocolate when you feel down?"
"How much tea/iced tea do you drink each day?"

## 5.25 Suicidal Behavior: (See also section 13.19 Suicide)

INITIAL INQUIRY:

"You have told me about some very painful experiences. They must have been hard to bear and perhaps you sometimes thought of quitting the struggle/hurting yourself or even killing yourself" If this idea is accepted by the client ask the about the following areas:

DEATH WISH:

"Has it crossed your mind that if you were to die that would end the pain you feel?"
"When was the last time you wished you were dead/thought you/others/the world would be better off if you were dead?"
"Have you thought this way before?"

IDEATION:

"When was the first time you thought of/considered ending it all/killing yourself?"
"When was the last time you thought of/considered ending it all/killing yourself?"
"Do you feel that you want to die now?"
"How often do you think of suicide? When you have suicidal thoughts how long do they last?"
"What brings on these thoughts?"
"How do you feel about these thoughts?"
"Do you feel you have control of these thoughts?"
"What stops/ends these thoughts?"

AFFECTS AND BEHAVIORS:

"How often have you felt lonely, felt fearful, or, because you you mood not eaten, slept poorly, gotten into a physical fight, or gotten drunk or high?"

MOTIVATION:

"Why are/were you thinking of killing yourself?"
"Have you felt "My life is a failure" or "My situation is hopeless?""
"What would happen after you were dead? What effect would your death have on others?"
"Under what conditions would you kill yourself?"

DETERRENTS/DEMOTIVATOR:

"What would prevent you from killing yourself?" (e.g. "I'm a coward; no courage", my children, religious convictions, shame, "I wouldn't give her the satisfaction")

GESTURE/ATTEMPT:

> "When was the first time you tried to kill yourself?" "How did you try?"
> "When was the last time you tried to kill yourself?"
> "Have you tried more than once?"
> "What were you thinking at the time about death or dying?"
> "Did you intend to die then?"
> "What happened before each attempt?" (an argument, conflicts with family, a humiliating experience, disappointments, school difficulties, incidents with police, a pregnancy, an assault, physical/sexual, you were told "I wish you would die")
> "What happened afterward?"(hospitalization (intensive care unit, psychiatric, general medical), effects on family and friends, on yourself, counseling or therapy?)

PLAN/MEANS/METHOD:

> "Have you made any plans to hurt or kill yourself?" [degree of detail]
> "How would you do it?" "Do you have the means?" [availability, opportunity]
> "Are you making preparations?" [collecting pills, loaded gun]
> "Have you written a suicide note?"
> "Have you given away any possessions of yours/written a will/checked on your insurance/made funeral arrangements?"
> "Have you told anyone about your plans?"

OTHER:
> "Has any relative or friend of yours ever tried or succeeded in killing him or herself?" (number, time when tried, most recent attempt)

# 6. Introduction to the Report and Identifying Information

## 6.1 The Evaluation:

Use a complete heading or stationery for identification of the evaluator by name, degree and title, agency affiliation, supervisor

Dates and location (e.g. in the hospital room, school's office, private office, home visit) of examination/ evaluation/interview(s)/testing, time of day, total time of testing.etc. as relevant.

ALWAYS date the report.

## 6.2 The Evaluation Process Consisted of:

Review of reports furnished/case histories/treatment summaries and reports/school records/previous evaluations, etc.

Interview with the client/friend/spouse/parents/family/care-giver/child

Testing - list separately each test by its full name and use abbreviations/acronyms in the body of the report.

Consultation with other professionals

Observational interview of the client/child/family

"All tests were administered, scored and interpreted by this report's author without the use of assistants or supervisees."

## 6.3 The Client:
The description should be so detailed as to enable the identification of the unique individual. (see section 8.0 Behavioral Observations)

Name: given, Christian, married, family of origin, maiden, changed, aliases

Identification: e.g. address, case number, client of ___ , etc.

Gender (not sex)

> **For a Child**: nickname(s), Prefers to be known as ...

Only as of demonstrable relevance:

> Age
>> **For a Child:** Use 9 years and 3 months, or 9  3/12, or 9' 3" not the ambiguous 9.3 years

> Marital status:
>> Current - never married (avoid "single" as it is ambiguous)/living with a partner/married, common law marriage/separated/divorcing/divorced/widow/widower/unknown
>> Number and duration of marriages, common-law marriages, separations, divorces, etc.
>>
>> [Note: Be consistent in reporting marital status data for both males and females]

> Occupation: employed/unemployed, other occupations, part-time work, previous occupations, etc. (see section 22.0 Vocational)

> Nationality/ethnicity, language used in the home

> Race: Black/African-American, white/Caucasian/"Anglo", Oriental, Hispanic, Latino, Native American, Inuit ("Eskimo"), Oceanic, Asian, etc., biracial/multiracial.
>
> [Note: Be consistent across reports in reporting race; do not report it only for minorities. If in doubt about a person's race or what are currently or personally acceptable terms, ask.]

> Residence/living circumstances: born into, recent if changed, current

> Religion: parental/baptized into/raised in/rejected/atheist/agnostic/non-practicing/unaffiliated/ unimportant to this person
>
>> Preference: converted to/practicing/devout/righteous/proselytizing/evangelizing/ preoccupied/delusional

## 6.4 Referral Reason:

Client was referred by ___ (referral source - person and agency)

On (date of referral)

For (rationale/purpose):

> for mental status evaluation, clinical interview, diagnostic determination, forensic evaluations, custody evaluation, pre-treatment evaluation and recommendations, educational placement, vocational recommendations, etc.

> (If no specific reason) ... to determine the nature and extent of psychiatric/psychological disabilities, assist with the development of a treatment/rehabilitation/education program, evaluate suitability for entry into ____ program, assess extent of neurological damage, determine benchmarks of current functioning, meet organizational needs for evaluation, assist with legal/forensic decisions, etc.

**For a child** (in alphabetical order):

| | | |
|---|---|---|
| Acceleration in grade | Aggressive behavior | Anxiety |
| Cheating | Compulsive talking | Daydreaming |
| Disruptive classroom behaviors | Dropping out | Drug abuse |
| Dysgraphia | Dyslexia | Difficulties with eating |
| Encopresis | Enuresis | Eye preference |
| Hand preference | Hyperactivity | Hypochondriasis |
| Idioglossia | Incontinence | Imaginary playmates/fantasy |
| Lying | Masturbation | Low motivation |
| Over-dependency | Nail biting | Phobias |
| Prejudice | Profanity/obscenity | Retention in grade |
| Running away | School phobia/avoidance | Sexual inappropriateness |
| Shyness | Sibling rivalry | Social isolation |
| Stealing | Temper tantrums | Thumb-sucking |
| Tics | Truancy | Underachievement |

(Modified from Attwell, Arthur A. (1972). *The school psychologist's handbook*. Los Angeles, CA: Western Psychological Services)

In preparation for/advance of the interview I received and reviewed the following records: ___ . Records were destroyed/unavailable/scant/unhelpful/scattered/adequate/pertinent/voluminous

I saw (name of client) on (date) (and total time and time of day if relevant) following your kind referral.

Legal mental health status: in/voluntary treatment/commitment, (give the number or name of the applicable section of the local law)

## 6.5 Complaint:

Patient's view of illness in his or her own words, and beliefs about the source(s) of the complaints.

Onset, circumstances of onset, triggers/cues/precipitates/stimulants

Duration, progression and severity of presenting complaint

Effects of the complaint on the functioning of the patient

Effects of treatments on complaint

Reasons and goals for seeking treatment at this time

Formal/chief/presenting complaint

Evaluator's clarification or reformulation or elaboration of complaint

**For a Child:** parental/teacher's/authority's perception of problem(s)

## 6.6 Other Aspects to be Considered at the Beginning of the Interview:

Ask about any need for glasses/contact lenses or hearing aids if not worn and comment on the effect or lack of degree of impairment on the client's performance.

Current medication prescribed/taken: Name(s), dosage(s), frequency

Handedness/preference/dominance (insert here or under section 8.4 Praxis)

## 6.7 Self-sufficiency in appearing for examination:

Came to first (or second, etc.) appointment, late by ___ minutes/excessively early/appropriately early for examination/on schedule/exactly on time for examination

Came alone or accompanied, role of companion in examination

Degree of difficulty finding the office

Drove/driven/mode of transportation

## 6.8 Consent

Introduce yourself by name and title

Explain the purposes of the interview

Obtain clear consent

### INFORMED:

We discussed the evaluation/treatment procedures, what was expected of both the
client and the evaluator/therapist, who else would be involved or affected, the
treatment's risks and benefits, and alternative methods's sources and costs and
benefits.

The client knows that the results of this evaluation will be sent to ... and used for ....

In a continuing dialogue these have been explained in language appropriate to his/her
education and intellect.

S/he understands the procedures, their consequences/effects, alternative procedures
and their consequences, and the decisions involved which s/he is being asked
to consent to.

### VOLUNTARY:

S/he understands and willingly agrees to fully participate.

S/he understand that s/he may withdraw his/her consent at any time and discontinue
treatment.

### COMPETENCY TO CONSENT:

I have no reason to suspect that this person in not competent to consent to the evaluations/
procedures/treatments being considered.

S/he is not a minor, nor mentally defective, nor does s/he have any limitation of communication,
psychopathology or any other aspect which would compromise his/her understanding
and consent.

6.9 Reliability/trustworthiness: (see also section 12.0 Standard Statements for an ABNORMAL Mental Status Evaluation Report )

RELIABILITY:

On the basis of
observations of this person for __ hours on __ occasions in (settings)
internal consistency of information and history
absence of omissions/deletions of negative information, contradictions
the character and cohesiveness of the client's responses, spontaneous comments, and behaviors
consistency of information from different sources
client's ability to report situations fully
the data/history are felt to be completely/quite/reasonably/rather/minimally/questionably reliable.

VALIDITY/REPRESENTATIVENESS:

Results are believed to be a valid sample of his/her current level of functioning/typical behavioral patterns/accurately represent his/her behavior outside the examination setting because he/she refused no test items/questions, he/she worked persistently/was most cooperative/had no interfering emotions such as anxiety or depression
Test findings/results of this evaluation are representative of his/her minimal/usual/optimal level of functioning
S/he attempted to be cooperative with the interview and indeed was helpful.

ACCURACY:

(<->) Complete/quite organized presentation/accurate recall of details/names and sequences/sparse data/stingy with information/only sketchy history/nebulous/vague/ambiguous/illogical contradictory
S/he presented personal history in a spontaneous fashion, organized in a chronological sequence and with sufficient detail, consistenty, and logic and attention.
Poor/adequate/good/excellent historian
His/her response to questions appeared to be free of any deliberate attempts to present a distorted picture.
Although somewhat dramatized, the core information appears to be accurate and valid for diagnostic/ evaluative purposes.

S/he had difficulty presenting historical material in a coherent and chronological manner.
The information offered is disorganized/haphazard/factitious/scattered.
S/he becomes tangential when pressed for specifics.

She/he tries hard to be accurate in recalling events but ....
She/he tried to provide meaningful responses to my questions but ....

The history offered should be taken with a grain of salt/was fabricated/grandiose
Was a willfully poor historian
Ganser's syndrome/hysterical pseudodementia/*vorbeireden*

TRUSTWORTHINESS

She/he seemed to be honest in her/his self-descriptions of her/his strengths and weaknesses.
Her/his appraisals tended to be supported by my observations.
S/he appeared to be a truthful witness and an accurate historian.
I believe s/he has been honest/truthful/factual/accurate.

# 7. Background Information
This section consists of many areas of HISTORY and ADJUSTMENT

## 7.1 History/Course of the Present Complaint/Problem/Illness: (see also section 6.5 Complaint)

Onset date and circumstances, precipitating stresses/situation, pre-morbid personality and functioning levels, development of signs/symptoms/behavioral changes, longitudinal/chronological/biographical sequence, periods of/attempts to work/return to functioning since onset, current status

## 7.2 Pertinent Medical History or Findings:

PSYCHIATRIC:

    Psychological difficulties in the past, treatment(s)/professional help sought
    Hospitalizations: date(s), name(s), location(s), condition on admission(s), therapies instituted and response to treatment(s), duration(s) of hospitalization(s), condition on discharge(s), time(s) before next hospitalization, intercurrent illnesses
    Current and past medications/therapies/treatments received, effects of/response to/treatments, side effects, condition(s) on discharge(s) from treatment
    Remissions:
        therapeutic, spontaneous
        duration
        return to what level of function/symptomatology: decompensation/damage/recompensation/recovery/adjustment/overcompensation/growth
    Recurrences/exacerbations/worsenings/flare-ups

    Reason for current admission/is result of ....
    Suicide: ideation/gestures/attempts (see section 13.19 Suicide)
    Needed precautions: sexual misbehavior, suicide, elopement, assault, homicide

PREVIOUS TESTING OR EVALUATIONS:

    *Type:* History and Physical, neurological, intellectual, educational, neuropsychological, personality, projectives, organicity, vocational

    Availability, results/findings, scores, comparisons with current results, omissions and contradictions, "rule-out"s

PREVIOUS PSYCHOTHERAPY OR COUNSELING:

    Dates, nature of problems, providers and nature of services, outcome

## Background Info

MEDICAL:

> Childhood illnesses
> Symptoms (use a checklist such as the Symptom Check List-90 for completeness)
> Diseases/disorders with known psychological aspects, e.g. thyroid, Mitral Valve Prolapse, AIDS, diabetes, cancer of the pancreas, etc.
> Surgeries
> Pregnancies: gravida (#), para (#), abortio (#)
> Injuries/accidents: especially closed-head and unconsciousness-producing incidents
> Drug treatment, use and abuse, street/illegal/illicit drug use (see sections 5.23 and 13.18 Substance abuse)

## 7.3 Personal, Family and Social Histories and Current Social Situation:

FAMILY OF ORIGIN: [Construction of a genogram (see section 3.7 General Notes) may be useful to guide inquiries and to record findings]

### For a child:

> Present family problems: marital conflict, separation, death of a parent/sib, relative, criminal victimization, work difficulties, financial concerns, drug/alcohol abuse, medical illness, disabilities, etc.

PARENTS':

> Personality characteristics, manner of relating to client, disciplinary methods, client's perception of parent's influences
> Marriages and divorces, separations, severe illnesses
> Qualities of the marital relationship: stormy, close, distant, warm, functional, etc.
> Occupation(s), effects of employment/career on client
> General physical and mental health during client's childhood, present health, chronic illnesses, disabilities, obligations
> History of substance abuse or misuse, physical or sexual abuse, traumas
> Age/birth date/year and cause of death, client's age and reaction to death and its consequences

SIBS'/STEP-SIBLINGS'/HALF-SIBLINGS'

> Ages, sex, location in a birth order/sibline/sibship/confraternity/constellation of (#) of children/sibs/siblings, relationships among sibs in past and at present
> General physical and mental health during client's childhood, present health, chronic illnesses, disabilities

DEVELOPMENT AND HEALTH/MEDICAL HISTORY:

Pregnancy: product of an unplanned but accepted pregnancy, full term, premature by __ weeks, difficulties/illnesses before/during pregnancy

Delivery: natural/prepared/unprepared/difficult/uneventful/easy, duration of labor was __ hours, birth weight, Apgar scores, birth defects,

Exposure to toxins/drugs/alcohol/diseases/insults pre/peri-/post-natally

Development:
    Post-natal difficulties, weight gain, eating, sleeping, daily routines
    Milestones: timing/delays in development in _____ area(s)/advanced/gained and later lost, crawling, sitting up unaided, walking, toilet training, speech and language, immature behavior patterns

Present health situation: cough, runny nose, flu, illnesses, medication(s), handicapping conditions

SOCIAL SITUATION:

Living arrangements: both parents, step/remarried parents, single parent, grandparents(s), foster homes, institutions, relatives, adoption, lives with whom, relationship, language in the home, legal issues

Location: city/metropolitan/urban/suburban/rural/institutions/military bases

Home supports: destitute/homeless/poverty, working poor, welfare/Aid to Families with Dependent Children/Social Security (Supplemental Security Income, SS Disability Income)/working class/middle class/upper class, disrupted/consistent, many/few/no moves

Social relationships: many/few/no friends, close/best friends, organizational membership, cultural interests, friends/buddies/clique/peer group membership/ or isolation/exclusion/rejection/ "loner", (see also section 20 Social/Interpersonal Functioning)

ADULT SOCIAL HISTORY AND SITUATION:

Marriage(s): age/date/termination reason, number/age/sex of children, relationship with ex-spouse/spouse/children, adultery/extra-marital relations/exclusivity/monogamy

Current social setting: living circumstances: lives alone/with family/other persons/alone but with much family support

Vocational/occupational: (See also section 22 Vocational Evaluations)
    Previous job's nature/demands/durations
    Present occupation- chosen?, duration, satisfaction?, intellectual demands, social-behavioral requirements/demands

Military service: none/alternate service/avoided/enlisted/volunteer/draftee, training, work performed, promotions/demotions, branch, duration, adjustment, combat/combat zone/non-combat/location, reenlistments, length of service, final grade, kind of discharge

Legal/Criminal history: charges as a minor, warnings from police, charges/indictments, arrests, prosecutions, convictions, incarceration/probation/parole, civil suits, current litigation/lawsuits, bankruptcy, violence directed against anyone

Exposure history to toxins and risks

Other: special skills, career goals, debts/burdens/adequacy of income to meet responsibilities/needs (see also Section 22. Vocational)

Recreational activities (see section 23. Recreation)

# Background Info

SEXUAL HISTORY AND SITUATION: (see section 5.20 Sexual History)

SCHOOLING - PAST AND PRESENT:

    School is:
        pre-school/kindergarten/elementary/middle/junior high/high school/ 2 or 4 year college
        rural/suburban/urban/inner city
        day/full time/part time
        public/private/special (indicate needs met), parochial/religious/sectarian
    Teacher, relationship(s) with teacher(s), teacher's report/description of problems
    Class assignment/level: grade/freshman/sophomore/junior/senior, age-grade differential
    Regular classes, Special Education: Trainable Mentally Retarded, Educable Mentally Retarded,
        Learning Disability classes, Socially and Emotionally Disturbed, Mainstreamed, Scholar's
        program, Gifted in (subject(s))
    Overall level of academic achievement/performance/grades, Quality/Grade Point Average, standing in
        class, major area of study and its relationship to present employment
    Grades completed, "social promotion" or earned advancement, dropped out of school in grade (#) at
        the age of (#)
    Degree obtained:Academic/Technical/Vocational/ General Equivalency Degree/College Preparatory/
        etc.)
    Extracurricular activities, athletics, social service, music, scholarly, religious, political
    Are there behaviors inimical to the welfare of other pupils?

## 7.4 Typical Problems of Children at School: (see also section 13.1 Attention Deficit Disorder)

SOCIAL:

Clique membership/exclusion, fights with ___, isolates self, "different", doesn't belong,
Timid/shy/dependent/anxiety prone, is an object of scorn/ridicule/mockery/teasing/name-
    calling/threats/physical attacks
Attention seeking behaviors: tattling, baiting, lying, provoking others, overly demanding of attention
    from teachers/peers/adults, craves ___ 's attention
Interpersonal: (<->) refuses to complete work assignments, seldom prepared, unmotivated,
    reluctantly participates, requires 1:1 supervision, gets along/is accepted/valued as friend

COGNITIVE:

Distractible, inattentive, handles new or exciting situations poorly, lacks foresight, low frustration
    tolerance, gets confused in group, does not finish his/her work, daydreams, does not take
    responsibility for own work/belongings

BEHAVIORAL:

Slow moving or responding, lethargic, hypo-active, < normal > impulsive/hyperactive/overactive
Conduct disorder: uncooperative/non-compliant, oral aggression/resistant, disruptive,
    bullies/intimidates, teases, agitates students/disturbs/disrupts other kids, low respect for
    authority/confronts teachers/defiant, insults, defies, troublemaker, aggressive, steals, truant,
    expulsions/suspensions/disciplinary conferences

PHYSICAL:

Fine motor coordination: cuts, draws, ties, writes, dextrous, alternates right-left, ambidextrous
Gross motor coordination: walks, runs, jumps, hops, skips, climbs, balances, falls, catches

STUDENT'S PERCEPTIONS:

of grades, source of problems, other problems, fairness of system, attitude of peers/teachers/
    administrators

OTHER ASPECTS:

Behavior deteriorates when confronted by academic demands

## 7.5 Typical Problems of Children at Home:

SYMPTOMATIC: These are in alphabetical order as no theory provides an agreed upon structures. See also parallel parts of the adult symptoms listed in section 13.Abnormal Signs and Symptoms.

Abuse: physical, suspected, being investigated, confirmed, by whom/relationship, duration
Aggression: physical attacking/violence, repeated threats, throwing things, verbal aggression
Autistic withdrawal: lack of responsiveness to people, resistance to change in the environment
Disobedience, negativism, non-compliance, defiance of authority, persistent rule breaking, lying
Eating: appetite changes, pica, weight gain/loss, anorexia, bulimia, obesity
Elective mutism
Encopresis
Enuresis
Fire setting
Legal difficulties: shoplifts, truancy, runs away, roams the streets, hangs out with peers, steals
Need for __ degree of supervision at home over play/chores/schedule.
Parasomnias: refusing to go to bed, nightmares, night terrors, sleepwalking, excessive drowsiness, refusal to get out of bed
Self-abusive behavior: tatooing, self-mutilation, scarring, cutting, insertion of objects into the body, biting or hitting self, head banging
Sexual: molests or molestation, threatens, fondles, intercourse-oral/vaginal/anal/femoral, repeated/single episode/recurrent, inappropriate sexual behaviors, assault, rape, force used, damage, medical attention/surgery, school/family/Mental Health - Mental Retardation Center/Child Protective services/police/court interventions, sexual preoccupation
Speech difficulties, stuttering (see section 8.5 Speech)
Temper tantrums: falls to floor and bangs heels/head, breath holding episodes, throws objects, screams, weeps, destructive, duration, how handled (Time Out, spanking, ignored, punished, mocked)
Tics: involuntary rapid movements, noise or word productions

CHILD'S PERCEPTIONS OF:

The parent's role of disciplinarian: uses lectures/force/spankings/groundings/allowance reductions/privilege losses as a consequence irregularly/arbitrarily/regularly, with good/mixed/poor success at control
Feels closest to mother/father/sib/uncle/aunt/grandparent/no one in the family
Physical/sexual molestation/abuse
Any symptomatic behaviors or complaints

## Referral Reason (see section 6.4 Referral Reason and 6.5 Complaint)

## Sexual History - Non-Symptomatic (see section 5.20 Sexual History)

## Substance Abuse History (see section 5.23 Substance abuse)

## 7.6 Adjustment History:

IN EDUCATION/MILITARY SERVICE/OCCUPATION(S):

> Able to conform to social standards, hold employment, advance in a career, adjust to superiors/peers/co/fellow workers, schedules, work load and task changes

SEXUAL ADJUSTMENT: (see also section 5.20 Sexual history)

> Disturbed sexual performance/dysfunctions: loss of desire, inhibited arousal, primary/secondary/occasional impotence, fast/premature/delayed ejaculation, inhibited orgasm, dyspareunia, vaginismus
>
> History of physical and or sexual abuse, molestation, violence/victimization, traumas
>
> Orientation and object choice: celibate, "sex addict", heterosexual, homosexual, lesbian, bisexual, asexual, etc.
>
> Paraphilias: sexual minorities/variations/special interests: pedophilia, exhibitionism, voyeurism, sadism and masochism, zoophilia, frottage, bondage and domination/discipline domination and submission, fetishism, transvestism (TV), water sports/urolagnia, Greek (anal)/French (oral)/English (whipping) sex, transexualism, etc.

SOCIAL ADJUSTMENT:

> Acquaintances, clique membership/exclusion, friends, buddies, best friends, relationship with sibs/friends/enemies
>
> Able to adjust to marriages, child birth/parenthood, losses, aging, illness, health care/services/treatments

## 7.7 Other Aspects of the History:

SOURCES:

> History from client/spouse/family/advocate/etc., from records (specify which)

QUALITY OF HISTORY OFFERED: (see section 6.9 Reliability)

OTHER:

> S/he denied the presence of any environmental or circumstantial, precipitating or contributing event which could have thrown her/him out of balance/destabilized her/his normal adjustment
>
> S/he has a most unfortunate history.
>
> Has a history of having lived for (#) years in an agonizing/tormenting/abusive/sociopathic/criminal/chaotic/pathogenic family
>
> His/her history is remarkable only for ... (findings).
>
> The patient was not questioned about sexual preferences/orientation, history or interests.

YVONNE DAVIS

**Background Info**

Notes and Additions/Suggestions:

# 8. Behavioral Observations (including Speech)

*THIS SECTION* covers the following areas: APPEARANCE including clothing

MOVEMENT of any kind

SPEECH behaviors

How the client      RESPONDED TO THE EVALUATION INTERVIEW and how s/he

PRESENTED HIM/HERSELF in the examination

are covered *IN THE NEXT SECTION* 9.0 Interpersonal Behavior

## 8.1 Communication barriers present:

Near/farsightedness, astigmatism, cataracts, hemianopsia, blindness, etc. Totally/partially/not
compensated for with glasses
Hearing impairment: total/partial deafness in left/right/both ears compensated for/with aids/lip
reading/signing/total communication/American Sign Language
Impaired speech (see section 8.5 Speech)
Unfamiliarity with the English language

## 8.2 Physical Appearance:
Note: Because, in the American culture, physical beauty is so tightly associated with goodness and health and
so impactful on a person's life course all clinicians should be fully informed of its consequences and
cautiously circumspect.

OVERALL APPEARANCE:

Hygiene is managed independently, effectively and appropriately.
No unusual physical features, unremarkable, clean, well groomed, well dressed
In No Apparent Distress

Appears older/younger than chronological/stated age
His/her appearance is not unusual. S/he would not be identified as unusual in a group situation on the
basis of physical appearance alone.
Disfigured, maimed, disabled, crippled

**For a Child:**
Appears to be well cared for/well trained in self care/assisted/supervised/ignored/neglected

BUILD: (<->)

| Emaciated | Thin | Average | stocky |
|-----------|------|---------|--------|
| sickly | lean | well-developed/built | chubby |
| malnourished | wiry | weight proportionate | heavy set |
| under-nourished | slender | to height | husky |
| underweight | lanky | well nourished | heavy |
| cachectic | skinny | within usual range | robust |
|  | bony | healthy | chunky |
|  |  |  | portly |
|  | petite | large-boned | beefy |
|  | diminutive | rangy | overweight |
|  | small-boned | large-framed | pot-bellied |
|  |  | rugged | formidable |
|  |  |  | hulking |
|  |  |  | enormous |

Height: It is preferable to state height objectively rather than in the "short/average/tall" relative terms.

Weight: Ask: "What do you now weigh?" and "Is this your usual weight?"

Note: Obese: "hardly/mildly/moderately/extremely/massively/morbidly" are all misleadingly subjective and subject to changing tastes and styles. It is far more preferable to report measured height, weight and general "build" or to weigh the person, and look in the Metropolitan Life Insurance Company's Table of Desirable Weights and report, say, "10% overweight."

**For a Child:**

Stature in relation to age is short/normal/tall, at the __ percentile of the standard tables for height and weight for children, Tanner stage (of sexual development) #

COMPLEXION:

Dark/light skinned/complected, swarthy, olive-skinned, florid, ruddy, red-faced, peaches-and-cream, tanned, sunburned, mottled, wan, sallow, jaundiced, sickly, pale, pallid/pallorous, leathery, weather-beaten, worn, wrinkled, pimply, warty, scarred, poorly complected

FACE:

Pinched, puffy, washed out, emaciated, old/young looking for chronological/true age, baby-faced, long-faced, moon-faced, dark circles under eyes, bulbous/red/richly veined nose
Movement: tics, twitches, drooping, mobility during interview/over topics
Notable features - ears, nose, cheeks, mouth, lips, teeth, chin, neck

✓ FACIAL EXPRESSIONS: (see also section 10. Affective symptoms)

Attentive, alert, tense, worried, indrawn, frightened
Sad, frowns, downcast, in pain, grimaces in pain, forlorn
Tearful/watered/tears up/tears falling/open crying/sobbing
Apathetic, preoccupied, inattentive, withdrawn, vacuous, vacant, absent, detached, mask-like, did not
    smile during the long interview, lacks spontaneous/appropriate/expected facial expression,
    flat, expressionless, lifeless, frozen, rigid, head bobbed as if nodding off
Calm, composed, relaxed, dreamy
Smiling, cheerful, happy, delighted, silly/sheepish grin
Angry, disgusted, distrust, contempt, defiance, sneering, scowling, grim, dour, tight-lipped, hatch
    marks between his/her eyes, has a chronic sour look

EYES: (see also section 8.4 Eye Contact)

Large, small, close-set, slanted, sunken, bloodshot, bleary-eyed, bulging, cross-eyed, "wall-eyed",
    staring, unblinking, glassy-eyed, vacant, penetrating, vigilant, nervously/frequent blinking,
    darting, squinting, tired, eyes twinkled, unusual,

Brows: beetling brows, massive, raised, pulled together, pulled down

Glasses: regular corrective lenses, half lenses, bifocals, reading glasses, contact lenses, sunglasses,
    needed but not worn, broken/poorly repaired

HAIR:

Hairstyle: of a fashionable length and style, long, pony-tail, pig-tails, corn-rows, braided, crew/brush
    cut, natural/"Afro", frizzy, curly, wavy, straight, uncombed, tousled, Punk, Mohawk,
    pageboy, currently popular haircut, unusual hair cut/style/treatment, moused, permed,
    relaxed, unbarbered, unremarkable
Color: bleached, colored/dyed, frosted, streaks of color, different color roots, salt-and-pepper,
    gray/color, faded color, fair-haired/blonde/platinum, brunette, brown, auburn, chestnut,
    black, red haired, albino
Other: Clean, dirty, unkempt, greasy/oily, matted.
    Thinning, receding hairline, high forehead, widow's peak, male pattern baldness, balding,
        bald spot, bald, head shaven, alopecia
    Wig, toupee, hairpiece, "a rug", implants, transplants, an obvious hairpiece
Beard: clean-shaven, unshaven/needs a shave, had the beginnings of a beard, whispy, scraggly,
    stubble, cultivated/deliberate stubble, grizzled, poorly/well maintained/groomed, neatly
    trimmed, full, closely trimmed, mutton chops, Goatee, Van Dyke/ZZ Tops/Santa Claus style
Moustache: wore/sported a moustache/moustached/moustacioed, oriental, handlebars, pencil thin,
    neat, scraggly, just starting

OTHER ASPECTS OF APPEARANCE:

Grooming: hygiene, cleanliness (excellent/good/unremarkable/fair/marginal/poor/awful), haggard, scruffy, unremarkable/as expected, neglected, acceptable but not optimal, neat, tidy, meticulous

Odor: body or clothing, musty, noticeable, offensive body odor, excess perfume, smells of alcohol

Teeth: unremarkable hygiene, dentures, gaps and missing teeth, edentulous, unusual dentistry, bad breath/breath odor/"halitosis"

Nails: cleanliness, tobacco-stained, dirty, grimy, bitten down to the quick, overlong, broken, polished, manicured

Skin: bruises, cuts, abrasions, scabs, sores, damage, tattoos, acne, *acne vulgaris* scars, scars, Port-wine stains, mottled

Head: odd shaped, microcephalic, macrocephalic, dolichocephalic, brachycephalic, normal, cretinous, damaged

Other: jewelry (rings, earrings, bracelets, pins, etc.), makeup, hearing aid, prosthesis, colostomy, catheter, other device

Notable aspects: shoulders, chest, breasts, back, pelvis, genitals, legs, feet, hands, fingers, swollen/wasted ankles/hands/parts

Breathing: noisy, wheezed, Shortness Of Breath, assisted, usual

BEARING:

Suggests chronic illness, appeared weak/frail, low stamina/endurance/easily winded, listless, labored, burdened, erect, "military", proud/arrogant, overly proper, deferential

OTHER STATEMENTS:

Shows some signs of self-neglect.

Shows the ravages of drug/alcohol/illness/stress/over-work/age/disease, dissipated, ill-looking, out of shape, tired, pathetic, pale and wan, frail, sickly

His/her personal grooming and hygiene while relatively neat and clean does reflect impoverishment/ very limited resources/cultural background/physical limitations/cognitive limitations.

## 8.3 Clothing:

APPROPRIATENESS: (<->)

For situation/occasion/weather, nothing unusual for a visit to a professional appointment/office

Presentable, acceptable, suitable, appearance and dress appropriate for age and occupation, business-like, professional appearance, nothing was attention-drawing, modestly attired

His/her idea of suitable, not suitable for age/suitable for a younger person, not suitable for his/her station in life, too casual to be acceptable, care of person and clothing was only fair

(<->) Institutional, odd, unusual, eccentric, peculiar, unique combinations, carefully disordered, dressed to offend, un/conventional, attention seeking/drawing, outlandish, garish, bizarre

QUALITIES OF CLOTHING: (<->)

| | | | | | |
|---|---|---|---|---|---|
| filthy | seedy | needing repair | plain | neat | stylish |
| grimy | disheveled | threadbare | out of date | careful | immaculate |
| dirty | neglected | rumpled | old-fashioned | dresser | meticulous |
| smelly | wrong size | clean but worn | old | overdressed | dandified |
| dusty | slovenly | worn | | clothes | elegant |
| oily | unkempt | shabby | | conscious | natty |
| greasy | ill-fitting | tattered | | in good taste | fashionable |
| food spotted | messy | unbuttoned | | | |
| | torn | unzipped | | | seductive |
| | sloppy | musty smelling | | regional/ | revealing |
| | baggy | | | foreign | flashy |
| | bedraggled | | | designs | too tight- |
| | raggedy | | | eccentric | fitting |
| | | | | | tasteless |
| | | | | | design |

OTHER:

Somber in hue, presents an employable appearance, shows unilateral neglect, overly prim
Dressed in a manner typical of today's youth/of the 1940's/1950's/1960's

# 8.4 Movement/Activity:

SPEED/ACTIVITY LEVEL: (<->)

Almost motionless, little animation, psychomotor retardation, slowed, slowed reaction time to
questions/latency, < normal >, restless, squirming, fidgety, fretful, constant hand
movements, hyperactive, agitated

**For a Child:**
Activity level: motoricly active, fidgets, difficult to redirect/redirectable, difficulty remaining in
his/her chair/seat, many out-of-chairs, restless and distractible, investigated all the
contents of the room/desk/testing materials, overactive/hyperactive/aggressive

COORDINATED/UNCOORDINATED: (<->)

Awkward, clumsy, inaccurate/ineffective movements, jerky, uncoordinated, < normal >, purposeful,
dextrous, graceful, agile, nimble
Degree of body awareness, body ego, body confidence

**For a Child:**
Coordination: delayed by __ months/years, gross and fine motor, noticeably poor manual
dexterity, held objects such as pencils awkwardly, difficulty coordinating hands and
fingers when asked to copy designs, hands were shaky on tasks

# Beh. Observations

PRAXIS:

>Handedness/preference/dominance
>Ask client to walk, write a sentence, tie shoes/tie.
>*Handshake:* (<->) Avoided, fishy, moist/sweaty/nervous, limp, tentative, delayed, normal, firm,
>    exaggerated, painfully tight
>Astereognosis

### For a Child:

>Grip: The student held the pencil in a grip considered correct/improper/in a fist-like
>    grip/atypical/awkward/in a palmar grasp/perpendicular to the table/down by the
>    graphite/with fingers too close to the point/thumb overlapping the forefinger/forefinger
>    overlapping the thumb/with two fingers and the thumb/with three fingers and
>    thumb/between the forefinger and third finger
>Slight problems in fine motor coordination were noted in making wavy/irregular/straight/
>    heavy/light/wild/uncontrolled lines.

MANNERISMS: (see also Symptomatic movements, below)

>Oddities of motor behavior/use of hands/body: rocking, aimless/stereotyped/repetitious/unproductive/
>    counter-productive movements, wriggles, bounces leg, posturing, hand or finger movements,
>    repetitive movements, covered face with hands and peeked out, engaged in self-stimulation,
>    hand flapping, walking on tiptoe/heels, made faces/grimaced, made odd/animal/grunting
>    sounds
>Manneristic mouth movements such as tongue chewing, lip smacking, whistling
>Yawned excessively/regularly/elaborately, appeared sleepy/tired, rubbed eyes
>Subtle signals, belching, picks/pulls at clothing, pulls lips into mouth
>Childlike gestures/facial expressions/speech (e.g. "Gol-lee")
>Sniffles repeatedly/loudly, uses/needs but does not use tissues/handkerchief, freely and frequently
>    picks his/her nose, repetitively "cleans" ears with fingers
>Made audible breathing sounds, whispered to him/herself

>Pauses and repeats movements at choice points as when leaving the room/in doorway
>Smoked incessantly/carelessly/dangerously/compulsively/selfishly
>Effeminate, overly feminine, mannish, "macho/a"

SYMPTOMATIC MOVEMENTS:

>Waxy flexibility *(cerea flexibilitas)*, tardive dyskinesia, dysiadochokinesia, Parkinsonian/Extra-
>    Pyramidal Symptoms/movements, athetoid, athetotic, akathesias, choreiform, akinesia, "pill-
>    rolling", "chewing", "Restless Leg Syndrome", opened and closed legs repeatedly, paced,
>    restlessness, hyper/hypotonic, hyper/hypokinetic, automatisms, command automatisms,
>    echopraxia, cataplexy, denudative behavior
>Tremor: none/mild/at rest/of intent/familial, quivers, shivers, twitches, tics, shakes
>Autonomic hyperactivity (see section 10.3 Anxiety)

MOBILITY: (<->)

>Confined to bed, bedfast, uses wheelchair, adaptive equipment, requires support/assistance/
>    supervision, uses a gait aid (cane, brace/leg/back, walker, crutches/Canadian, wheelchair,
>    geriatric chair), slow, careful, avoids obstacles

GAIT and STATION: (<->)

> Atasia-abasia, shuffles, desultory, effortful, dilatory, stiff, awry, limps, drags/favors one leg, awkward, walks with slight posturing, lumbering, leans, lurching, ataxic, collides with objects/persons, broad-based, knock-kneed, bow-legged, < normal >, ambled, no visible problem/no abnormality of gait or station, fully mobile including stairs, springy, graceful, glides, brisk/energetic, limber
>
> Mincing, exaggerated, strides, dramatic, unusual, able to locomote and navigate under his/her own power

**For a Child:**

> Uncoordinated, e.g. difficulty climbing stairs, brushed ankles against each other, unsteady forward gait, stumbled at intervals. (Note the wear patterns on shoes)

BALANCE:

> Dizzy, vertigo, staggers, sways, fearful of falling/unsure, unsteady, positive Romberg sign, complains of light-headedness, < normal >, no danger of falling, steady

POSTURE: (<->)

> Hunkered down, hunched over, slumped, slouched, stooped, round-shouldered, limp, cataplexy, relaxed, < normal >, stiff, tense, guarded, rigid, erect, upright, sat on edge of chair, odd, leans, peculiar posturing

EYE CONTACT: (<->)

> None, avoided, stared into space, stared without bodily movements or other expressions, kept eyes downcast, broken off as soon as made, passing, wary, alert, looked only to one side, brief flashes, fleeting, furtive, appropriate, effective, < normal >, expected, modulated, lingering, staring, glared, penetrating, piercing, confrontative, challenging

OTHER:

> Pain behavior accompanying movements: degree of difficulty getting down into and up from a chair, sighs, groans, grimaces, winces, braces, sits/walks rigidly, splinting (see also section 25.4 Chronic Pain personality)

**For a Child:**

> Dominance: mixed, right/left, as seen in hopping on a foot/preferred hand/use of one eye to sight/flipping a coin/catching a thrown object

## 8.5 Speech Behavior: Give quotes/verbatim/examples (see also section 8.6 Speech reflecting cognition)

ARTICULATION:

Unintelligible, stammer/stutter, stumbles over words, mumbles, mutters under breath, lisp, sibilance, slurred, juicy, garbled, understandable, clear, clipped, choppy and mechanical, poor diction, poor enunciation, pace/cadence/rate, too slow/fast, rhythm, accent, drawl, burr, misarticulated, unclear, dysfluencies, dysarthrias (spastic, flaccid, ataxic), aphasias

### For a Child:
Immature: simpler sentences/formation than expected, articulation errors, difficulty in speech articulation: especially sounds such as r, sh, th, z or ch

VOICE'S QUALITIES:

Loud/noisy/almost screaming, brassy, gravelly, hoarse, throaty, raspy, screechy, shrill, staccato, strident, harsh, mellifluous, quiet, soft, weak, frail, thin, "small" voice, whispered, affected, tremulous, quavery, low/high pitched, nasal, sing-song, odd inflection/intonation, monotonous tone, sad/low tone of voice, muffled

PHRASEOLOGY: (see also Content below)

Spoke in almost "babytalk"/infantile/childish/immature style, mispronounced words, uneducated vocabulary, uncultured language, slang words, grammatical mistakes, dialect, regionalisms, provincialisms, foreign words, idioms, cliches, habitual expressions, repetition of catch phrases, many "You know"s, pedantic, pseudo-intellectual, stilted, jargon, contrived, punning, rhyming, anomia, agramatism

### For a Child:
Underdeveloped vocabulary for his/her age
Conversation consisted of 3-4 word phrases rather than sentences

SPEECH AMOUNT/ENERGY/FLOW/RATE/PRODUCTIVITY: (<->)

| halting | Slowed | Normal | Pressured | Verbose Flight of ideas |
|---|---|---|---|---|
| hesitant | minimal response | initiates | loquacious | over-prod- |
| delays/ed | unspontaneous | alert | garrulous | uctive |
| inhibited | unresponsive | productive | rapid | bombastic |
| blocking | terse | animated | excessive | non-stop |
| | sluggish | talkative | wordy | vociferous |
| | paucity | fluent | exaggerated | over-abundant |
| | sparse | well-spoken | hurried | over-responsive |
| | hesitant | easy | voluble | |
| mute | laconic | spontaneous | voluminous | |
| elective | impoverished | smooth | talkative | |
| mutism | difficulty gener- | crisp | excessive detail | |
| | ating thoughts | even | expansive | |
| | taciturn | | blurts out | |
| word-finding | | | rushed | |
| difficulties | | | run-together | |
| word searching | | | raucous | |

MANNER:

| | | | |
|---|---|---|---|
| distant | normal | candid | empathic |
| hurried | warm | open | touching |
| pedantic | sincere | frank | insightful |
| somber | well modulated | guileless | wise |
| inarticulate | articulate | free | charming |
| whiney | gets ideas across well | untroubled | witty |
| | good natured | easy | jovial |
| expressionless | engaging | | |
| monotone | well-spoken | | |
| mechanical | eloquent | | |
| | realistic | | |
| | measured | | |
| | thoughtful | | |
| | responsive | | |

## 8.6 Speech as a Reflection of Cognition:

CONTINUITY: (<->)

| Incoherent | Loose | Idiosyncratic | disconnected | Clear |
|---|---|---|---|---|
| incomprehensible | circumstantial | unusual | topic changes | realistic |
| clang associations | irrelevancies | associations | difficult to | rational |
| neologisms | tangential | personal | follow | lucid |
| word salad | vague | meanings | fragmented | consistent |
| confabulations | derailed | poorly defined | perplexing | coherent |
| verbigerations | rambling | conjectural | flighty | relevant |
| perseverative | garbled | preoccupied | confusing | integrated |
| chaotic | confused | | unclear | goal- |
| | sidetracked | | mushy thinking | directed |
| | evasive | | intricate | logical |
| | distracted | | Byzantine | pertinent |
| | digressive | | baffling | easy to |
| | circumlocutions | | incorrect | follow |
| | paraphrases | | conclusions | intact |
| | word substitutions | | indefinite | sequential |
| | non-sequential | | | not pre- |
| | jumbled | | | occ- |
| | illogical | | | upied |
| | circular | | | |

# Beh. Observations

CONTENT: (see also section 13.3 Delusions, contents of)

| | | | | |
|---|---|---|---|---|
| personalized | trivial | obscene | over-detailed | self-critical |
| idiosyncratic | platitudes | profane | preoccupations | self-doubting |
| eccentric | empty | scatological | obsessions | ambivalences |
| odd | oversimple | sexual | over-valued ideas | |
| selective | | earthy | magical thinking | injustices |
| carefully chosen | | vulgarities | | plaintive |
| sentimental | life situation | pornographic | homicide | accusatory |
| flowery | stressors | impolite | running away | regrets |
| philosophical | illnesses | blasphemous | escape | tragedies |
| | disabilities | sexual | violence | frustrations |
| | family/relatives | | self-destruction | |

SUMMARY STATEMENTS FOR SPEECH: (see also section 12.7 Stream of thought)

*Normal:*

No language impairment receptively or expressively
Communication was not impeded in any way, satisfactory/adequate/normal expressiveness
No abnormalities of audition/hearing
Without articulatory deficit
Comprehension of English/spoken words was normal/defective/abnormal.
His/her ability to understand the spoken word was adequate within the context of this examination but
    might not be in ___
Auditory comprehension was adequate and oral delivery was effective.
His/her speech was sophisticated with considerable emphasis on intellectual/personal/medical/
    historical/family matters


Speech was relevant and appropriate and without evidence of unusual ideation
No impairment reflective of disordered mentation
There was a normal flow of ideas/continuity
His/her associations were well organized
Shows good grammatical complexity
His/her logic was easy to follow although the responses were superficial

S/he is a reciprocal conversationalist/dialogued spontaneously/is able to carry on a conversation
S/he is able to initiate topics appropriately.
S/he follows the conventions/social rules of communication including appropriate phrasing, turn-
    taking, and understood the suppositions and expectations of native speakers of American
    English

*Abnormal:*

Hearing was normal/normal with use of hearing aid/hard of hearing/partially deaf/read my
lips/required me to raise my voice/shout/completely deaf

Participated/did not engage in appropriate social dialogue
Little/normal/expected/excessive small talk

Does little analytic or discriminatory thinking
Converses in response to questions rather than speaking spontaneously, self sufficient in providing
responses but volunteered little additional information, would not enlarge/expand on topics of
interest, little/no elaboration of responses to my questions

Modulations/shifts of anxiety were inconsistent and unrelated to to the content or affective significance
of what s/he was saying

Word retrieval deficits/reports "forgetting"/has difficulty finding words/groped for words, sudden
stopping in mid-sentence/speech
Great difficulty gathering thoughts rather than in finding words
Substituted related words approximating the definitive/appropriate term
Paraphrasic errors, dysnomias, unusual word and sentence formations, errors of syntax,
constructional dyspraxia, malapropisms

When interrupted became confused and rambled

Assumed that I, the listener, knew more than I did about his/her history/ideas/the subject of the
conversation
Speech was slow, deliberate and, at times, evasive
All of his/her speech was defensive/designed to emphasize his/her degree of disability
His/her answers were not to be relied upon, but were pertinent and to the point. (see section 6.9
Reliability)
Uses vulgarity/blasphemy/scatology/sexuality to shock
Preoccupied (see section 12.7 Preoccupations)
Rote re-telling of an often-told story

**For a Child:**
Perseverative, echolalic, delayed language acquisition, difficulty in comprehending or
expressing oral language

## 8.7 Other Behavioral Observations:

NORMAL:

> Took good care of his/her appearance in regard to dress, hygiene, and grooming
> Nothing unusual/remarkable/noticeable about his/her posture, bearing, manner, or hygiene.
> No deformities

ABNORMAL:

> Brought to the examination: possessions, cigarettes, presents, papers, briefcase, coffee/refreshments/candy/food
> Fidgety, nervous and inappropriate laughter/smiling, titters, giggles, nervous habits. (see also section 10.3 Anxiety)
> Audible sighs, tearful, tears, crying, sobbing, hand wringing (see also section 10.4 Depression)

### For a Child:
> Tantrum: assaultive, destructive to property, aggressive to others, redirectable

# 9. Interpersonal Behavior

This section describes FACE-TO-FACE or one-on-one BEHAVIORS. For BEHAVIOR IN GROUPS see section 20. Social Functioning.

This section consists of two areas:    1. BEHAVIORS-IN-THE-EXAMINATION including
    RESPONSE to the PROCEDURES of evaluation
    RAPPORT
    RESPONSE to the METHODS of evaluation
    CONCENTRATION, MOTIVATION, RESPONSE TO
    FAILURE, and APPROACH
  2. SELF-PRESENTATION of the client to the evaluator.

## 9.1 Relating to the Evaluation Procedures (<->) (see also sections 9.2 Rapport , 9.4 Effort/ Attention/Concentration, and 8.5 Speech)

Unable to recognize the purposes of the interview/the report to be made, unaware of the social conventions, did not understand or adapt to the testing situation, s/he was not able to comprehend or respond to questions designed to elicit ____ or symptoms of ___, low attending skills, just able to meet the minimum requirements for appropriate social interaction, misconstrues what is said to him/her, unaware, unresponsive, echolalic, preoccupied, estranged, doesn't grasp essence or goal

    Dependent, sought/required much support/reassurance/guidance/encouragement from the examiner, desperate for assistance, self-doubting, ill at ease

        Indifferent, bland, detached, distant, uninvolved, uncaring, haphazard, insensitive, tense, bored, showed the presence of an interfering emotion, needed coaxing, over-cautious, related obliquely

            Anxiety appropriate/proportionate to the interview situation, initially responded only to questions but later became more spontaneous. Began interview with an elevated level of anxiety which decreased as the evaluation progressed. Needed assistance to get started.

                Understands the social graces/norms/expectations/conventions/demand characteristics of the examination situation, comfortable, confident, relaxed, interested, curious, eager, intense, carefully monitored the testing situation, oriented, aware, alert, cooperative, no abnormalities, attends, responds, reciprocates, continues, participates, initiates, communicates effectively, clear and efficient, high quality of interaction, with depth

**Interpersonal  Behs.**

> **For  a  Child:**
>
>> Behavior when with parent:
>>> Played easily in the waiting room [level of play, put away the toys used, age
>>>> appropriate playthings]
>>>
>>> Control used by parent [degree, kind/methods/means, timing, over issues of _____ ]
>>> Relationship, supportive, agreed to?
>>> Parents agreement/disagreement/conflict on discipline
>>
>> Separation from parent: degree and type of anxiety, coping mechanisms used on separation,
>>> the parent(s) management of separation was ...
>>
>> S/he was reluctant to separate from her/his parent/accompany the examiner to/into the interview
>>> room, came willingly into the examination/testing room/office with the examiner,
>>> accompanies the examiner easily/readily, separates easily/poorly/reluctantly from the
>>> examiner, resists returning to parent, comfortable with adults, masters own anxiety,
>>> needs much reassurance, responded well to reassurance, reaction upon rejoining
>>> parent, easily redirected or distracted from parent
>>
>> Parental interaction with examiner
>>> Attitude/type of relating: arrogant, suspicious, cooperative, trusting, dependent
>>>> controling/manipulative, seductive, dependent, impatient, threatening
>>>
>>> Role taken and role assigned to examiner, changes during interview
>>
>> Feelings aroused by child in examiner
>
> **For  an  Adolescent:**
>
>> Limited spontaneity which was not inappropriate for his/her age.

## 9.2 Rapport/Relationship to Examiner:

COOPERATION/POSITIVE BEHAVIORS: (<->)

| | | | | |
|---|---|---|---|---|
| affable | Cooperative | Dependent | Indifferent | seductive |
| pleasant | helpful | institutionalized | no effort | immature |
| friendly | easy to interview | agreeableness | frustrated | practical |
| chummy | enjoyed | deferential | docile | joker |
| outgoing | interview | ingratiating | passive | clowns |
| socially | | trying to please | sedated | exhibitionistic |
| graceful | without hes- | eager to please | submissive | |
| solicitous | itation | effusive | lackadaisical | |
| tactful | responsive | obsequious | doesn't try | |
| cordial | answers readily | pleading | accommo- | curt |
| gracious | obliging | over-solicitous | dating | monosyllabic |
| amiable | agreeable | | minimal | legalistic |
| warm | amicable | obedient | cooper- | passive agg- |
| familiar | | confidential | ation | ressive or |
| genial | | conciliatory | sheepish | dependent |
| jokes around | | oily | | |
| breezy | | fawning | noncommittal | |
| playful | courteous | flattering | compliant | |
| easy | well-mannered | | blasé | |
| inoffensive | polite | defers | careless | snippy |
| "laid back" | civil | humble | nonchalant | sassy |
| low key | | over-polite | | flippant |
| "mellow" | | over-apologetic | | spooky |
| placid | | eulogistic | | |
| | | apple-polishing | | "forgets" |
| frank | | mealy-mouthed | | |
| forthright | | plaintive | | |
| candid | | help-seeking | | |
| | | barters affection | | |
| | | wants to please | | |

# Interpersonal Behs.

RESISTANCE/NEGATIVE BEHAVIORS: (<->) (see also section 10.2 Anger for emotions)

| Guarded | Surly | Defensive | Demanding | Hostile | Argumentative | Belligerent |
|---|---|---|---|---|---|---|
| reserved | sulky | subtle | imposing | irritating | territorial | insulting |
| reticent | petulant | hostility | insistent | instigating | possessive | defiant |
| recalcitrant | balky | uncooperative | indignant | obnoxious | antagonistic | obstreper- |
| resistive | touchy | "sick and | confrontative | tests limits | contentious | ous |
| reluctant | pouty | tired" | presumptuous | derogatory | oppositional | scolding |
| inaccessible | sullen | non-compliant | frustrated | loathes | manipulative | |
| distant | brooding | | complaining | | provocative | |
| remote | crabby | | domineering | | quibbles | |
| evasive | testy | | rebellious | | questions | name-call- |
| wary | gruff | | rude | | hypercritical | ing |
| withdraws | snappish | | nagging | | irascible | vilifying |
| withholding | peevish | | resentful | Superior | quarrel- | slandering |
| avoidant | grouchy | | | pities | some | menacing |
| not forth- | scowls | | Stubborn | distant | | venomous |
| coming | "snippy" | | mulish | aloof | sarcastic | threatening |
| tight-lipped | | | intractable | disdainful | abusive | nasty |
| | Childish | | unbending | egocentric | derisive | malicious |
| suspicious | immature | | unyielding | entitled | scornful | caustic |
| cagey | uncertain | | unadaptable | cocky | sarcastic | |
| sneaky | | | rigid | over-bearing | carping | |
| | | | obtuse | arrogant | berating | |
| over-controlled | | | inflexible | contemptuous | | |
| businesslike | | | negativistic | supercilious | facetious | |
| stiff | | | abrasive | toyed with | mocking | |
| unfriendly | | | opinionated | examiner | taunting | |
| desultory | | | willful | "knows-it-all" | sneering | |
| habit-bound | | | contrary | smart-alecky | smug | |
| | | | cantankerous | | | |

OTHER STATEMENTS: (see also section 9.8 Social Presentation)

Rapport was easily/intermittently/never established and maintained
Response to authority was cooperative/respectful/appropriate/productive//indifferent/hostile/
    challenging/unproductive/non-compliant, poor attitude toward authority.
Required/allowed another to answer none/some/all of the questions posed

Was cooperative within limits; s/he refused some test items/tests/topics
Was fully cooperative with the examiner only after determining my credentials
Gave only perfunctory/superficial cooperation
Responded slowly/gave purposefully erroneous responses as a form of resistance, performed half-
    heartedly, showed minimal compliance
Repeatedly/irrelevantly/provocatively interrupted the interviewer

He/she appeared to be feigning cheerfulness/good spirits.
The testing/questions/history taking/examination was particularly trying for him/her

I could easily understand his/her meanings. S/he was open, available

EYE CONTACT: see section 8.4 Eye Contact

## 9.3 Response to the Methods of Evaluation/Tests/Questions

COMPREHENSION OF INSTRUCTIONS/QUESTIONS: (<->)

Rarely understands instructions, requires much repetition/elaboration, needed to have instructions repeated often, gets confused, required restructuring of my questions in a manner to make them more concrete and simplistic

> May sometimes need elaboration of instructions, attentive, understands, good comprehension, required excessive time and repetition to understand what was required of him/her

> > Quickly grasps problem, anticipates the response expected/desired

APPROACH/ATTACK/STRATEGY: (<->) (see also Summary Statements, later)

| Random impulsive | Indifferent giggled flippant | Scattered inconsistent careless disorganized sloppy uncoordinated | Organized coordinated controlled goal-oriented active diligent | Rigid compuls- ive ritualistic persever- ative |
| --- | --- | --- | --- | --- |
| distracted agitated | | | catches on fast well-ordered | perfection- istic |
| Distrusts own ability | Haphazard acts without instructions | Baffled | thinks through before acting | manner- istic |
| self-doubting | non-plussed | | notes details     tense | |
| second guesses self | thinks aloud | | uses trial-and- | |
| insecure | absent-minded | | error approach | |
| unsure | guesses at | | orderly | |
| refuses to guess | answers | | methodical | |
| /take chances | | | deliberate | |
| underestimates | Hurried | | persistent | |
| own abilities | fast | | neat | |
| | rapid | | contemplative | |
| | speedy | | pensive | |
| | rushed | | matter-of-fact | |
| | | | thoughtful | |

## 9.4 Effort/Attention/Concentration: (<->) (see also 8.5 Speech, Amount)

| | | | | |
|---|---|---|---|---|
| Apathetic | Sluggish | Distractible | Normal energy | Eager |
| dull | worked slowly | low attending skills | cooperative | animated |
| uninvolved | in slow motion | easily distracted | interested | fascinated |
| uninvested | slow reactions |   from task | adequate | |
| passive | slowed | loses concentration | good effort | initiates |
| anergic | | does not stick | spontaneous | inquisitive |
| | Reticent |   with task | open | enthusias- |
| listless | unspontaneous | had great difficulty | attentive |   tic |
| bored | taciturn |   following directions | alert | well- |
| disinterested | | non-persistent | |   spoken |
| inattentive | Flat | | | verbal |
| bland | no originality | | | garrulous |
| exhausted | unchanging | | | eager to |
| tired | expressionless | | |   ventilate |
| listless | uncreative | | | talkative |
| indifferent | paucity of | | | |
| shuns effort |   worthwhile ideas | | | candid |
| resigned | | | | in touch |
| | | | | with own |
| Inconsistent | Perplexed | | |   feelings |
| skimpy responses | baffled | | | |
| sporadic | bewildered | | | dramatic |
| varies with task | confused | | | over- |
| | uninformed | | |   abundant |

## 9.5 Motivation/Persistence/Perseverance: (<->)

Refuses test items/subtests, only brief responses, had to be prompted to elaborate, gives up on easy items, seeks to terminate interview, quits quickly, gives up easily

Variable level of interest/motivation, slowed/varying reaction time to questions, needs frequent/constant reinforcement/encouragement/reassurance/praise/commendation for continued performance, sustained effort only for ___ time period, often discouraged, low frustration tolerance, prefers only easy tasks, little tolerance for ambiguity, initially refused to attempt tasks but upon re-presentation later was cooperative

Withdraws, shows irritation/anger, complains, refuses

Accepts own inferior performance, satisfied with inadequate work, inimal concern and care about doing well on evaluations, no motivation to succeed with difficult tasks/perform well for the examiner, took breaks and recovered willingness to continue, began to lose interest in the evaluation tasks and in conversing with the examiner after ___ time.

Average perseverance and effort demonstrated, only rarely discouraged or inattentive

Changes tasks appropriately, eager to continue, challenged by difficult tasks, concentrates on one task for a long time, finishes every task, distracted only by extreme circumstances, sustains effort, persists, diligent, wanted to do well

## 9.6 Response to Failure/Criticism/Feedback on test items and Self-awareness/Self-monitoring/Self-criticism (see also section 9.2 Rapport) (<->)

Oblivious to failure, no response to either success or failure, unaware of/unconcerned about/failed to recognize errors, examiner's questions/suggestions/hints didn't improve performance, low self-monitoring/error correction skills, hypocritical, inappropriately over-confident

Flustered, embarrassed, ashamed, chagrined, apologetic, self-reproaches, self-derogates, feelings are easily hurt, rationalizes failures, extremely critical of work/hypercritical

Normal responsiveness and coping with failure, tries his/her best, surprised at failure, accepts mistakes with regret, accepts need to go on despite failure/mistake/incorrect answers, confident, calm, understands easily, adapts, modulates, good balance of self-criticism and self-confidence, self-sufficient, learns from errors/experience, accepts own limitations so failure has little effect

Self-congratulatory, proud, delighted with success, persists, works harder, self-monitors, sought errors in own work and self-corrected, gives up only on items clearly beyond ability, refuses to concede defeat, wasn't discouraged by errors, was easily motivated by "Try again"

**For a Child:**

Clapped/squealed with satisfaction/excitement/delight
Seemed to enjoy the opportunity to talk openly with the professional

## 9.7 Other Statements about Approach/Attack/Strategy, Task Performance, Attention, Attitude, Motivation, Persistence and Response to Criticism:

PRODUCTIVE:

Consistent and organized
Waited for full instructions
Listened attentively to the interviewer's questions
No problems with test directions or instructions
His/her understanding of the spoken word was good; directions/'instructions did not have to be
    repeated or rephrased/simplified
Only repetition/slowed presentation, not simplification, of test directions was required
Was able to follow multi-step directions

Fully responded to all tasks' demands
Applied him/herself to the tasks presented
Organized his/her ideas before responding to test questions
Was cooperative and put forth best effort on each evaluation task administered
Became quite involved in the tasks
Participated well and fully in the evaluation process
Willingly/eagerly attempted each task presented
Testing seemed to be challenging and interesting to him/her

Adequate attention span, concentration, little distractibility, anxiety or frustration
The source of distractions were ... and he/she was successfully able to resist distraction by ....
Demonstrated no negative attitudes

S/he related each presented test item to some direct experience in his/her own life.
Asked relevant/insightful/helpful questions
Stepped back and reviewed behavior when s/he failed; did not stick with an obviously ineffective
    approach.

COUNTER/NON-PRODUCTIVE:

S/he terminated effort following minimal concentration
Perseverated in that he /she had difficulty adjusting and responding appropriately to the next task's
    demands/instructions

Took a great deal of time, longer/shorter than usual reaction time/latency of response to questions
Worked at an even pace throughout regardless of task at hand

Showed the long-term effects of defective innate ability, low expectations, an unstimulating
    environment, and poor/minimal formal training
His/her performance was depressed by poor application of skills he/she does already possess/by
    fatigue
Marginal approach to the evaluation reflective of ...
    mildly/moderately/severely reduced intellectual capacity
    poorly developed cognitive strategies
    generalized undisciplined mental processing
    lack of self evaluation/little concern for the quality of his/her responses.
Impulsive responses with poor organization and planning skills, without forethought, minimal
    reflection/consideration before answering

# Interpersonal Behs.

S/he was not task oriented

Used avoidance techniques in examination such as dropping test materials, starting conversations between subtests, attending to sounds in the hallway, asking repeated questions regarding the test materials and procedures, wandering off-task

When the test materials became necessarily too difficult s/he became frustrated and wanted to give up

Used random trial and error approach on most tasks and showed little comprehension, visualization or analysis of the overall tasks, little learning from his/her attempts

S/he is not flexible in problem approaches/lacks problem attack skills/perseverates manner of problem attack

Stresses details but misses main point/"can't see the forest for the trees"/doesn't "catch on"/"misses the boat"

Defective performance was present only on items which ... and not on items/areas of ...

Had difficulty answering questions but cooperated to the best of his/her ability

Tried to provide meaningful answers to specific questions but no additional information was forthcoming.

S/he was frank with his/her answers but could not give detailed information.

He/she was unaware of the low level at which he/she performed

Efforts at compensation through ___ (e.g. a pedantic style) create a negative impression of which s/he is apparently unaware

His/her perception of his/her status and abilities are somewhat inflated

S/he is not so skillful as he/she thinks

Tried to have the examiner confirm one of a number of offered responses as the correct one

Answered almost all questions with "I don't know"

Invariably responded with "I don't know" to questions but, on repetition of the question produced a good/correct/scoreable response

## For a Child:

When asked questions in his/her mother's presence he often/always/rarely glanced at/turned to her hoping she would answer the question/seeking confirmation of his answer/deferring to her superior knowledge.

Very resistive behavior: (<->)
> Uncontrollable, destructive, untestable, acting out, temper tantrums, disruptive of testing, unruly, distractible, difficult to evaluate, difficult to handle, stubborn

Counts on fingers

Covered his face with his hands

Looked about the room but was redirectable

# 9.8 Social Presentation

PRESENCE: (<->)

| | | | | |
|---|---|---|---|---|
| Withdrawn | Shy | Threatened | Self-assured | autonomous |
| isolating | timid | distrustful | friendly | direct |
| estranged | aloof | fearful | inviting | dominant |
| distant | passive | plaintive | jocular | surgent |
| suspicious | sheltered | reticent | warm | business-like |
| guarded | dependent | vulnerable | outgoing | assertive |
| asocial | | weak | jolly | |
| introverted | Reserved | delicate | extraverted | stubborn |
| solitary | retiring | would crumble | chipper | insistent |
| seclusive | humble | fragile | animated | |
| detached | subdued | distraught | engaging | |
| | bashful | threat-sensitive | charming | |
| dejected | introverted | unspontaneous | | |
| | restrained | | | |
| | mild mannered | | | |
| | composed | | | |
| | placid | | | |

DEPENDENCY/SURGENCY: (<->) (see also Presence, above)

Spineless, meek, servile, timid, clinging, whining, suppliant, tenuous, tentative, frightened, docile, defers, inoffensive, passive, yielding, acquiescent, amenable, "wishy-washy", compliant, assenting, consenting, cooperative, independent, dominant, forceful, masterful, high-handed, autocratic, dictatorial, blustery, pugnacious, over-bearing, pushy, demanding, exaggerated sense of own importance, has "hutzpah"

SOCIAL SOPHISTICATION: (<->)

Unsophisticated, gullible, naive, wide-eyed, suggestible, "Pollyanna"-like, "Little Orphan Annie", "positive thinking", forced optimism, uneducated, unschooled, backward, inept, culturally unsophisticated, medically/psychologically naive, simple, simplistic, immature, passive, giddy, flighty, lacking in self-sufficiency, socially immature, naive attempts at manipulation, guileless, over-used "Yes, M'am/Sir" and "No, M'am/Sir"

Mannerly, polite, graceful, poised, "finesses"

Sophisticated, socially skilled, cultured, street-smart, seductive, articulate, able to lobby/defend his/her interests

Blunt, tactless, pointed, provocative, abrasive, offensive, vulgar, rude, offered outspoken criticisms

Opportunistic, manipulative, sociopathic, callous, predatory, "innocent"/blames others, general denial, irresponsible

# Interpersonal Behs.

WARMTH: (see also 9.2 Rapport - Cooperation) (<->)

      Over-indulgent, doting, affectionate, affable, tender, gentle, sympathetic, friendly, gracious, kindly, outgoing, considerate, convivial, companionable, intimate, gentle, genteel, sweet, soft-hearted, saccharine, oily, phoney

SELF-IMAGE/SELF-ESTEEM: (See also Confidence, below)

      Self concept, identity, body image, body ego, personal space, property, sex role, sexual identity, age identity and role, confidence, self esteem, autonomy, goals for self

CONFIDENCE: (<->)

      Expresses an exaggerated opinion of him/herself, believes s/he is exceptionally capable despite evidence to the contrary, self-exalting, boastful, vain, cocky, pompous, conceited, confident, self-respecting, modest, unassuming, humble, self-doubting, self-deprecatory, self-abasing, describes self as "a loser/failure/misfit"

OTHER ASPECTS OF CHARACTER/PRESENTATION OF SELF/DEMEANOR:

      Is self-contained and in good charge of him/herself, reserved, collected, matter of fact, static, mechanical, stereotyped, rigid, expressionless, stoic toward his/her illness/limitations

      Prim and proper, straight-laced, prudish, dour, austere, prissy, "stuffed shirt", self-righteous, puritanical, rigid
      Admits to the compulsive virtues of neatness, orderliness, and planning ahead
      Pious, sanctimonious, over-religious, Bible-centered life, Church-centered lifestyle

      Childish, immature, juvenile, backward, silly, childish attention seeking, his/her manner is suggestive of a much younger person, suggestive of a person much younger emotionally than physically,

      "Nerdy", socially unskilled/inept, preoccupied with irrelevancies
      Dull, simple-minded, "air-head", vapid, insipid
      Inattentive, stares, forgetful, preoccupied, mind elsewhere, "space cadet", "Spacey", "Zombie-like", "burned out"

      Begging, pleading, coaxing, needy
      Presented him/herself as frail and inadequate person of whom one should not expect much

      Embarrassed/ashamed/self-blaming/self-reproaching/guilty, "worthless"
      Worrisome, a "worry wart" or excessive worrier, easily threatened, inept, feelings are easily hurt, manifested anxiety throughout the interview around every topic
      Became apprehensive when talking of behavior s/he now realizes was inappropriate

      Exaggerated, flamboyant, dramatic, melodramatic, theatrical, histrionic
      His/her somatic complaints are unusual, even singular, and were described in affect laden terms

      Vivacious, bubbly, volatile, labile, pert
      Over-sexualized: saucy, coy, titillating, suggestive, flirtatious, girlish, boyish

Bragging, cocky, tended to praise him/herself excessively, mildly antisocial manner, cavalier
Assumed/maintained an attitude of tolerant amusement.
His manner was swaggering in order to impress the interviewer with his youthfulness/energy/
       toughness.
Client uses embellishments and attempts to appear as a) a "bad actor" or powerful and dangerous
       person e.g. uses vulgarity to shock, presents as a "tough cookie" or, as b) possessing a high
       potential, or many friends, etc.

A "character", individualistic, idiosyncratic, "marches to his/her own drummer", unusual ways of
       perceiving/behaving, eccentric, "oddball", does not fit in, outlandish, flamboyant, strange,
       odd, peculiar, bizarre, weird

Menacing, frightening, imposing, awesome, intimidating, manipulating, "Spooky", vaguely but
       intensely frightening, enjoys sadistic humor/is prankish

Intellectualizes: provides psychological jargon/"psychobabble"/labels when asked for descriptions of
       behaviors/symptoms.

Recites life as a series of mishaps, melodramatically enumerates life's misfortunes, made a saga of
       his/her life in the telling, offered a woeful tirade/Jeremiad of woes/baleful stories/ "Oliver
       Twist" like story, presented her/himself as a "Born Loser" or perpetual victim or outcast

Client puts up a good front to cover ...
Was reluctant to expand on/denies her/his complaints/problems/symptoms

Offered little information but responded readily to direct questions
Was very verbal but not articulate
Where one word would suffice/answer the question asked s/he produced a paragraph
Attempts to be helpful by trying to tell a great deal and so creates pressured speech
S/he made sure to tell me what s/he thought I should hear and know and then it seemed that s/he felt
       satisfied
S/he indicated a sense of righteous entitlement to his/her ... (e.g. alcoholism, violence,
       irresponsibility, etc.)

Clock-watched
Offered/desired inappropriate bodily contacts
Focused on the Examiner's office/accent/clothing/manner/role/appearance rather than the content of
       his/her/my speech or point of the interview

Client was questioned extensively and creatively but it was not possible to determine/get a clear
       picture of/more information on _____
Responded eagerly to leading questions endorsing the presence of symptoms or problems if
       suggested
Impossible to obtain any delineation of symptoms other than his/her informal description of"I lost it"
Despite allegations of pain and deficiency he is able to get up and down from a chair without difficulty

Client is deliberately deceptive, malingering, faking good/bad
Motivated only to obtain benefits/malingering.
Client's attitude toward his/her illness/disability suggests indifference/tolerance/acceptance/
       transcendence

## Interpersonal Behs.

There are no obvious physical or behavioral stigmata which would set him/her apart from other
individuals of his/her age, social or cultural group
S/he put forth good effort to collaborate in the evaluation
S/he is aware of the social norms and is able to conform to them
Knows/utilizes/obeys the rules of conversation and turn-taking
His/her responses reflect wishful thinking rather than realistic plans
S/he is dependent on institutional support and content to be hospitalized/taken care of

## For a Child:

Pseudo-mature, uncommonly independent
Primitive, socially inappropriate, non-aggressive behavior
Attitude and feelings toward:
    Clinic visits: grasp of purpose, awareness of own difficulties, reaction to symptoms, feelings
        about returning to clinic
    Self: behavior, appearance, body, sex, intellect, worries, fears, preoccupations
    Others: parents, sibs, school, peers, authorities
Playing observed:
    Plays with same/younger/older age peers
    Approach and interest in toys, materials, toys actually used
    Mode of play: incorporative, extrusive, intrusive
    Manner of play: constructive, disorganized, mutual, distractible, disruptive

---

## Speech and Verbal Interactions: (see sections 8.5 Speech and section 9.2 Rapport)

---

## Reliability: (see section 6.9 Reliability)

# 10. Emotional/Affective Symptoms and Disorders
After the general statements about affects emotions are presented in alphabetical order.

## 10.1 Mood and Affects:
Mood is usually considered to be a self-report (but sometimes an inference) of pervasive and sustained emotional coloring of one's experience, a persistent emotional trend (like the climate). Affect is of shorter duration, such as what the clinician observes during the interview, and is more variable and reactive (like the weather). Note and document any differences between the two during the interview.

BEHAVIOR reflecting emotional state:

> Tears, flushing, movements (tremor, etc.), respiratory changes and irregularities, voice changes, facial expression and coloring, wording, somatic expression of affects through ...

Give quotes/self report of mood/affect/emotion

### General aspects of Mood and Affects:

GEOGRAPHY:

> Elevated/flat/depressed

SOURCE:

> Reactive, endogenous, exogenous, characterological

AMOUNT/RESPONSIVENESS/RANGE: (<->)

| Flat | Blunted[1] | Constricted | Appropriate | Broad |
|------|-----------|-------------|-------------|-------|
| affectless | restricted | contained | integrated | deep |
| bland | restricted in range | low intensity | euthymic | intense |
| unresponsive | inexpressive | shallow | responsive | generalized |
| vacant stare | expressionless | muted | normal range | pervasive |
| | unchanging | subdued | supple | |
| | | "low key" | | |
| | | detached | | |

CONGRUENCE:

> Appropriateness/incongruous to situation and thought content, face reflects the emotions reported, all were thoughts colored by emotional state, indifferent to problems, floated over his/her real problems and limitations, *la belle indifference*

DEGREE:

> Mildly/moderately/severely/profoundly... (E.g. depressed)

---

[1] Consider the possible effects of current medications

DURATION/MOOD CHANGES: (<->)

> Mercurial/quicksilver, volatile, affective incontinence, dramatic, excitable, transient, unstable, rapid mood fluctuation, labile, fluctuates, plastic, changeable, moodswings, flexible, appropriate, diurnal/seasonal mood cycles, long cycles, shifts in tension, mobility of emotional state, consistent, showed little/normal/much variation in emotions, frozen, permanent

EPISODE OF AFFECT DISORDER:

> Initial, single, sporadic, episodic, repetitive, recurrent, cyclical, seasonal, annual, anniversary reactions, exacerbated, chronic, in remission

> Recurrent episodes appear to be worsening as the depression is more severe, longer/shorter symptom-free periods, periods of improvement are to a lower level, and medication produces slower/less improvement

---

## 10.2 Anger: (see also section 9.2 Rapport - Resistance for more Behavioral aspects)

GENERAL ASPECTS:

> Sources of, intensity, direction, target, handling, coping methods, impulse control

HOSTILITY/VERBAL HOSTILITY/INDIRECT ANGER: (mood and affects) (<->):

| | | | |
|---|---|---|---|
| Irritated | Temperamental | Hostile | Shouts |
| annoyed | whining | provoked | furious |
| disgruntled | restive | embittered | threatens |
| cranky | piqued | exasperated | enraged |
| miffed | "pissed off" | indignant | incensed |
| displeased | "burned up" | simmering | choleric |
| sullen | "bugged" | seething | bellicose |
| ill-tempered | bothered | | infuriated |
| bad-tempered | | | |
| grudging | | | |
| brooding | | | |

VIOLENCE/AGGRESSION/BEHAVIORS: (see section 13.11 Impulse control)

## 10.3 Anxiety:

AUTONOMIC NERVOUS SYSTEM: (over-arousal) facets of Anxiety:

| | | | | |
|---|---|---|---|---|
| Pallor or flushing | Shortness Of Breath | Dizziness | Clamminess | Trembling |
| | chest tightness | unsteadiness | hot flashes | shaking |
| Heart palpitations | chest pain | vertigo | sweaty palms | jitteriness |
| fast heartbeat/racing | choking/smothering | room spinning | cold sweats | jumpiness |
| | fast respiration | light-headedness | excessive perspiration | muscle |
| | hyperventilation | faintness | sweaty-forehead | aches |
| Diarrhea | | syncope | dry heaves | |
| frequent urination | Paraesthesias | | dry mouth | |
| stomach churned | | voice cracks | | |
| | | voice tremor | | |

BEHAVIORAL FACETS OF ANXIETY:

"Nervous habits" (<->)

| | | | |
|---|---|---|---|
| self-grooming | Can't sit still | Unable to proceed | Panicked |
| scratching | leg swinging | unable to function | rushed out |
| fidgeting | rocking | immobilized | vomited |
| restlessness | pacing | rigid posture | fainted |
| fretful | stretching | inhibited movements | |
| muscle tension | self-hugging | sits on edge of chair | |
| wringing hands | | | |
| clutching hands | | Erratic | |
| worried look | Coughing | jumpy | |
| scratching | nail biting | oversensitive | |
| yawning/sighing | flashes of smiles | to stimuli | |
| strained voice | tears/crying | over-reactive | |
| tremulous | wide-eyed | easily startled | |
| agitated | brow grooves | | |
| tapping | | | |
| repetitive movements | | | |

AFFECTIVE FACETS OF ANXIETY: (<->)

| | | | | |
|---|---|---|---|---|
| Terrified | Fearful | "Nervous" | Calm | Imperturbable |
| horrified | apprehensive | uneasy | phlegmatic | stolid |
| rigid | frightened | harried | steady | |
| panic attacks | alarmed | | unemotional | |
| panicky | | vulnerable | stable | |
| frozen | "uptight" | fragile | composed | |
| petrified | a "worrier" | tense | nonchalant | |
| paralyzed | "a worry wart" | edgy | "cool" | |
| | | "on edge" | confident | |
| | | frazzled | | |
| | | flighty | | |

**Affective Sx**

Cognitive facets of Anxiety: (<->)

> Baffled, confused, ruminative, perplexed, bemused, upset by fantasies/imagined scenarios/criticisms/ attacks/hurts, ill at ease, overwhelmed, having a cascade of symptoms, sense of impending doom, apprehensive, worrisome, uneasy, guilt-ridden, perfectionistic, secure, assured, eager, unconcerned

Interpersonal facets of Anxiety: (See also section 9.8 Presence)

> Thin-skinned, easily threatened/aroused to anxiousness, insecure, vulnerable, oversensitive, self-conscious, timid, timorous, uncertain what to say or how to act

Anxiety: *(subjective):*

> High internal tension, feels inept, nervous, can't handle stress/pressure/demands, vulnerable, low self-confidence/efficacy, confused, indecisive, insecure, "fluttery", "quivery", "feels like I'll explode/my heart will burst through my chest"

Anxiety: *(Inferred):*

> No depth of feeling when recounting events, erratic, guardedness, rigidity, confuses self, self-induced pressures, jumps from one subject/topic to another, low frustration tolerance, low stress tolerance, low tolerance for ambiguity, impulsive/acts out

Other statements:

> Shifts in anxiety level during interview not/related to subjects of discussion

## 10.4 Depression:

### *Affective facets of Depression*

ANHEDONIA:

> Abscence of pleasure, apathy, boredom, loss of pleasure in living, "nothing tastes good anymore", joylessness, lack of satisfaction in previously valued activities, loss of interests, no desire/energy to do anything, no fun in his/her life
>
> Indifference, "couldn't care less", lowered or no desires, nothing good to look forward to in life

DYSPHORIA:  (<->)

| | | | | |
|---|---|---|---|---|
| Wretched | Melancholy | sadness | petulant | moody |
| inconsolable | despondent | blue | whining | |
| anguished | gloomy | "down in the | plaintive | |
| suicidal | dejected | dumps" | | |
| miserable | sorrowful | beaten down | | |
| desperate | forlorn | glum | | |
| pathetic | bitter | tearful | | |
| worn out | dysphoric | doleful | | |
| drained | morose | dour | | |
| exhausted | funereal | cheerless | | |
| in pain | despairing | somber | | |
| suffering | disconsolate | downcast | | |
| | grave | gloomy outlook | | |
| | profoundly sad | "down" | | |
| | woeful | "wiped out" | | |
| | profoundly unhappy | troubled | | |
| | morbid | | | |
| | somber | | | |

### *Behavioral facets of Depression:* Vegetative signs/physical malfunctioning:

SLEEP PATTERNS: (See also section 13.16 Sleep disturbances)

> Early Morning Awakening, terminal insomnia, hyposomnia, hypersomnia, asomnia, reversal of day/night cycle, Sleep Continuity Disturbance, restless sleep

EATING:

> Appetite increase or decrease, fewer/more frequent meals, fasting, pica, selective hungers, binges, weight increase or decrease

PSYCHO-MOTOR RETARDATION/ACCELERATION: (see also section 8.4 Movement )

> Absence of/lessened spontaneous verbal/motor/emotional expressiveness, long reaction time to questions (indicate number of seconds), repetition/urging needed, thoughts stop/slowed/laborious/impoverished/racing
> Wrings hands, rubs forehead, shuffling gait
> Little inflection, flat/expressionless/monotonous voice

**Affective  Sx**

LIBIDO: (sexual interest, not activity) (see section 5.20 Sexuality)

BOWEL/BLADDER HABIT CHANGES

> Diarrhea/constipation, increased frequency of urination, over-concern with elimination, chronic use or abuse of laxatives, sensations of abdominal distention or incomplete evacuation

OVER-USE OF

> Prescription and over-the-counter medications (analgesics, laxatives, sleeping aids, vitamins), alcohol, e.g. caffeine

APPEARANCE:

> Sad/fixed/expressionless/unsmiling facies, downcast face, distracted look, blank stare, furrowed brow, audible sighs
> Close to tears/tearful/teary, tears well up, weepy/weeps, cries, blubbers, sobs,
>
> Dissipated, worn, drained, "a shell of a person", haphazard slef-care

ENERGY:

> Lowered energy, slowed down, listless, "needs to be pushed to get things done", "everything is an effort", easy fatigue, tired, feels "run down", mopes, weakened, lethargic, de-energized, torpid, anergia, lassitude, "can't shake off the blues", energy is just adequate for life's tasks, drained, exhausted

OTHER:

> Diurnal variation, depression's symptoms are worse in morning and lessen as day wears on
> Suicidal ideation (see section 13.19 Suicide)

## Cognitive facets of depression

CARING/ENERGY INVESTMENT:

| | | | |
|---|---|---|---|
| Hopeless | Pessimistic | cold | Bored |
| helpless | suspicious | unconcerned | indifferent |
| cynical | disappointed | stoic | lethargic |
| unchangeable | disillusioned | phlegmatic | apathetic |
| nihilistic | skeptical | | ennui |
| defeated | resigned | | |
| futile | discouraged | | |
| negative | demoralized | | |
| bleak | disenchanted | | |
| feeling lost | defeatist | | |
| colorless | loss of ambition | | |
| dreary | goalessness | | |

MENTAL DULLNESS:  (<->)

| | | | |
|---|---|---|---|
| inadequate | slowed | confused | empty |
| unable to cope | indecisive | perplexed | unclear |
| frustrated | excessive worrying | matter-of-fact | vague |
| | worrisome | worsened memory | meaningless |
| | ruminative | decreased concentration | lost |

## SELF-CRITICALNESS/BROODING: (<->)

| | | | | |
|---|---|---|---|---|
| vulnerable | regretful | ashamed | humiliated | cowed |
| self-doubting | sorry | self-reproaching | suppressed rage | awed |
| threat sensitive | chagrined | "a failure" | self-hating | over- |
| criticism-sensitive | self-blaming | "inferior" | self-abusing | whelmed |
| rejection-sensitive | self-depreciating | fault-finding | "worthless" | |
| self-pitying | embarrassed | self-critical | | |
| "poor me" | self-condemning | "useless" | | |
| low self-esteem | ineffectual | "a loser" | ironical | |
| self-distrusting | unproductive | "a freak" | sarcastic | |
| intimidated | "inadequate" | "wasted my life" | | |
| | | "a misfit" | | |

## SUMMARY STATEMENTS FOR COGNITIVE ASPECTS:

Demonstrated Beck's negative view of the self, world and future
Dwelt on past failures, lost opportunities, what could never be, roads not taken, etc
S/he needed time to mobilize/gather his/her thoughts
"feels like I'm here physically but not mentally/really present"
Distrusts own mind/thinking processes, feelings/guts
No plans for him/herself, no future, nothing to look forward to in life, only an empty repetition of
meaningless actions

## *Social facets of Depression*

### INTERPERSONAL: (<->)

| | | | | |
|---|---|---|---|---|
| Reclusive | Avoids people | distrustful | irritating | strained |
| inaccessible | distances | resentful | irritated | relationships |
| asocial | self-absorbed | argument- | bitter | dependent |
| barricades self away | withdraws | ative | demanding | passive |
| non-spontaneous | low social interest | suspicious | crabby | unassertive |
| hermit-like | subdued | feels scorned | easily irritated | wary |
| secludes | painfully shy | feels abandoned | easily annoyed | |
| isolates | separates from life/others | | arguementative | |

### SUPPORT-SEEKING: (<->)

Complains of life's unfairness, righteous, gossips, envious, gripes, futilely indignant, sympathy
seeking, whiney, self-pitying, manipulative, emotionally hungry, seeks support only when in
crisis, finds others always inadequately supportive or sympathetic

## *Other facets of Depression:*

S/he is depressed because forced into dependency by disability/losses/injury
Mirth response is spontaneous, excellent//normal/adequate/diminished/absent/sarcastic/ironical
Depression is worse during winter (consider Seasonal Affective Disorder)
Dexamethasone suppression test results supported ...

Suicide: (see section 13.19 Suicide)

## 10.5 Guilt: (<->)

Self-condemning, self-reproaching, penitent, begging forgiveness, repentant, pleading, sorry, at fault, ashamed, chagrined, regretful, contrite, remorseful, concerned, burdened, responsible, apologetic, cold, hardened, unreformed, cynical, unrepentant, conscienceless, shameless, unscrupulous, parasitic, incorrigible, predatory

## 10.6 Mania:

### AFFECTIVE FACETS OF MANIA: (<->)

| Labile | | unstable | rapid fluctuation | accelerating course | |
|--------|--------|----------|-------------------|---------------------|--------|
| Cheerful | High | Hypomanic | Exuberant | Manic | Ecstatic |
| light-hearted | gay | buoyant | elated | | exalted |
| positive | laughing | silly | ebullient | | rapturous |
| bright | buoyant | giddy | false joy | | euphoric |
| vivid | jovial | excessively cheerful | false elation | | |
| intense | elevated | boisterous | | | |

### BEHAVIORAL FACETS OF MANIA:

(<->) Fast/rapid speaking, overtalkative, overabundant, loud, verbose, garrulous, tirades, singing, rhyming, punning

(<->) Periods of hyperactivity/over-activity, paces, restless, speeded up, accelerated, quickened, fast, going fast, racing, frenzied, manic, assaultive

Overconfident, starts many activities but does not finish or follow through with most.

Insomnia, decreased need for sleep

Incautious, fearless, engaging in reckless activities e.g. dangerous driving, foolish business investments or buying sprees, impulsive spending, sexual indiscretions or acting out or greatly increased need for sexual activities, hypersexual, disinhibited activities, increased smoking, telephoning

### COGNITIVE FACETS OF MANIA: (<->) (see also 12.7 Stream of thought)

| | | | | |
|--------|--------|--------|--------|--------|
| Expansive | Grandiosity | Flight of ideas | loosened associations | delusions |
| word plays | pressured speech | illogical | disjointed | incoherent |
| ideas of | abrupt topic | racing thoughts | disorganized | bizarre |
| reference | changes | thought | disoriented | |
| hyperbole | idiosyncratic | bombardment | | |
| little or no insight | associations | brief attention span | Hallucinatory | |
| over-productive | | limited concentration | experiences | |
| exaggeration | | distractible | | |
| *witzelsucht* | | sexual/religious | | |
| frivolous | | preoccupations | | |

SOCIAL/INTERPERSONAL FACETS OF MANIA:

(<->) Impatient, intolerant, insulting, uncooperative, resistive, negativistic, critical, provocative, suspicious, angry, irritable, over-sensitive, touchy, easy/inappropriate anger, nasty, loud, abusive, crude, foul language, swears, curses, blasphemes, vulgar, bathroom language, obscene

Suspicious, guarded, distrustful, believes other collude against him/her, asserts that s/he was tricked into ..., denies validity or reality of all criticisms

Gregarious, likeable, dramatic, entertaining, pleasant, seductive, vivacious, cracks jokes, prankish insincere, naive, infantile, silly

Entitled, self-important, grandiose, cocksure, emphatic, self-confident, "hutzpah"

Dominating, controlling, boastful, challenging, surgent, conflicts with authority figures

DELUSIONS: (see section 13.3 Delusions )

Fantasies of romantic involvement, grandiose business plans

---

## 10.7 Sexuality (See section 5.20 for history questions and 7.6 for sexual adjustment and history)

ATTITUDES AND BEHAVIOR: (<->)

Disgusted, apathetic,  inhibited, ashamed, puritanical, prudish, prim, restrained,     passive, hesitant, permissive, romantic, amorous, erotic, sensual, assertive, passionate, seductive, over-active, soliciting, compulsive, demanding, lustful, lewd, wanton, aggressive, assaultive

Increased or decreased: desire, arousal, activity/relations, satisfaction, hypo/hypersexuality, reluctance to initiate, slow to respond, previously inhibited interests

Abstinent, celibate

# 10.8 Other Emotions:

SENSE OF HUMOR (<->):

> Cosmic, wry, deadpan, dry, ironic, sarcastic, sophisticated, gentle, mirthful, playful, joking, funny, teasing, wise cracks, mocks, silly, slap-stick, tells jokes, tells stories, puns, off-color jokes, inappropriate remarks excused as "just kidding", hostile, offensive, non-existent sense of humor, "stuffed shirt", humorless, inappropriate laughter

GRIEF:

> Distress, sorrow, gloom, anguish, despair, heartache, pain, woe, suffering, affliction, troubles
> Preoccupied with loss/loved one/consequences/memories, easily tearful, slowed thinking and responding with long latencies of response, stares into space
> Feels helpless, vulnerable, useless, lowered self-esteem
> Denial, anger, bargaining, acceptance, transcendence

PRIDE:

> Dignity, self-respect/esteem/regard/image, confidence, righteousness,

> Vanity, ego, airs, arrogance, conceit, condescension, narcissism (see also 25.11 Narcissistic personality)

EMBARRASSMENT/SHAME/HUMILIATION:

> Disgrace, reproached, depreciated, devalued, humbled

AMBIVALENCE;:

> Mixed feelings, conflicted, at cross purposes, "left hand doesn't know what right hand is doing", indecisive, can't decide/make up mind, stuck, alternates, "want and don't want it at same time"

# 10.9 Other Statements about Affects:

Her/his affect was brighter than one would expect from someone in her/his position in life.
S/he is experiencing mental turmoil/upset/distress.

# 11. Standard Statements for a NORMAL Mental Status Report

Reliability/Trustworthiness: See section 6.9 Reliability

## NORMAL Mental Status:

Note: Most readers of Mental Status reports prefer specific, observable, and behavioral descriptions rather than conclusions, labels, and summary words.

OVERALL STATEMENTS:

In No Acute Distress, in No Apparent Distress, Within Normal Limits, average, unremarkable, intact, nothing unusual, was alert and spontaneously verbal

No limitations in any of the domains assessed by this/these instruments/examinations.

No evidence/signs of a thought disorder, major affective, cognitive or behavioral disorder were elicited.

No abnormalities of thought, affect, or behavior, no gross abnormalities, nothing bizarre, no cognitive slippage. I did not find any unusual kinds of logic or strange associations.

No/obvious indications of psychosis or organicity, no hallucinations in any field

S/he experiences thoughts in a spontaneous and normal manner, lucid and coherent, no disordered mentation, mentation is intact

He/she is in full/partial/marginal/shaky remission.

I failed to elicit any symptomatic behaviors/indicants of previously described symptoms or disorders.

Based on current observations there is no decompensation, deterioration, or exacerbation of past conditions.

No drug no alcohol abuse/legal/psychiatric history of diagnosis or treatment

Based on behavior observed during the interview, I believe ....

In my professional judgement ....

# NORMAL Mental Status

*Cognitive Functioning:* (see also section 8.6 Speech as a reflection of cognition)

ORIENTATION:

Her/his sensorium was clear.
S/he was fully oriented times three/to time, place and person, times four/to things.

PRODUCTIVITY:

Showed an average amount of thoughts and they were neither speeded nor slowed/moved at a normal pace
Seems normal from the perspective of productivity, relevance, and coherence

THOUGHT CONTINUITY:

His/her thoughts were clear, coherent, well organized, goal-directed and relevant to the subject at hand.
S/he reached the goal of his/her thought processes without introducing any irrelevant material.
His/her train of thought was goal-directed, relevant, and logical.
His/her stream of thought was coherent, focussed, and without digressions, irrelevancies, disturbances of logic or bizarreness.
There was no tangentiality, circumstantiality, or distractibility.
Her/his replies answered questions appropriately.
S/he presented her/his thoughts in an appropriately paced, understandable and relevant fashion.

THOUGHT CONTENT:

No obsessions or phobias, ideas of reference, hallucinations, delusions, faulty perceptions, perceptual disturbance, misinterpretations of consensual reality, or psychotic distortions.
Not preoccupied with obsessions, phobias, or suicide.

ABSTRACTION:

He/she was able to form concepts well.
Handled ideas well and without concreteness
He/she was able to identify similarities, differences, and absurdities
Was able to analyze the meaning of simple proverbs, all at appropriate levels of abstraction
S/he could give me the deep meanings of the proverbs I offered
S/he was able to respond with an abstract relationship between pairs of terms/items I presented to her/him.
Had common sense, functional understanding of everyday objects

COMMUNICATION:

I noted no impairments in language functioning reflecting disordered mentation.
S/he could comprehend and carry out the test/evaluation instructions and tasks, and didn't misinterpret or misunderstand the test materials or questions.

MEMORY:

All components of memory are all grossly intact
S/he is able to recount personal history normally.
His/her remote, recent and immediate memories appear to be intact as far as I can determine without
    independent verification of the historical facts.

JUDGEMENT:

Responded appropriately to imaginary situations requiring social judgement/knowledge of the
    norms/usual rules and expectations of society.
S/he is a thoughtful person who understands the likely outcome of his/her behavior and thinks ahead.
Has common sense understandings, subscribes to the usual explanations of people's motivations

REALITY TESTING:

Intact, functional, not distorted by psychodynamics or psychopathology, perceives the social world
    as do most people, understands cause-effect links as do other people, shares common
    attributions of causality
Functional/adequate/good/extensive fund of knowledge, awareness of the external world.

## Affective functioning:

Shows a range of emotions/feelings and they are appropriate to the ideational content and
    circumstances
Emotional reactions were relevant to the thought content and situation
Euthymic
No difficulty in initiating, sustaining, and terminating emotional expression
Adequate level of emotional energy
His emotions seemed appropriate during the interview/examination. He was not depressed, elated,
    anxious, angry, or suspicious.

## Other statements:

Cognitive functioning seems limited rather than faulty
Showed a good balance of self-esteem/confidence and self-criticism
Precocious, very learnèd, brilliant
Cognitive style: global/impressionistic, field dependent/independent, leveler/sharpener, rigid/flexible

**NORMAL Mental Status**

Notes and Additions/Suggestions:

# 12. Standard Statements for an ABNORMAL Mental Status Report

As there is no consensus on the relationship of these components of cognition they are presented here in order of roughly increasing complexity of their performance.

## 12.1 Levels of Consciousness: (<->) (Use the Glasgow Coma Scale (Teasdale and Jenvet, 1974) for more precise numerical rating)

Coma, comatose, coma vigil, unarousable, unresponsive, obtunded

Stuporous, delirious, responsive only to persistent or noxious stimulation, post-ictal, twilight/dreamy state, drifts off, fluctuates, arousable/rousable, semi-coma

Lethargy, reduced wakefulness, somnolent, only briefly responsive with a return to unconsciousness

Clouded consciousness, drowsy, falls asleep, responding requires heightened effort, lessened ability to perform tasks, frequent hesitations, starting/startles, disoriented, groggy, "drugged", under the influence of medications which ...

Alert, responds to questions, attentive, makes eye-contact, interacts, asks questions, converses, alert, lucid, intact

## 12.2 Orientation:

Incorrectly identifies self by name, mistakes/confuses present location, correct time, objects, others, Mistakes/confuses dates/persons/places
Is off the mark by __ years/months/days
Oriented to ___ but not to ___
Oriented times/X three/four

## 12.3 Attention:

Unaware, unable to attend, inattentive, ignores questions, attention could not be gained nor held, attention limited by extraneous sounds/concurrent activities/fantasies/affects/memories

Distractible, attention wandered, attentive only to irrelevancies, responses are irrelevant, unable to reject interfering stimuli from environment/viscera/affects, guided by internal not external stimuli, easily overloaded by stimulation, cannot attend to coping/adaptive/purposeful tasks, cannot repeat familiar lists/phrases, attends only for brief intervals, can't absorb details needed for responsible judgements beyond the routine

Cannot follow a three stage command/written directions, cannot spell words forward and backward, preoccupied, selective attention, low attending skills, shows lapses of attention, redirectable

Focuses/selects the relevant among the irrelevant aspects of a situation, maintains the focus, resists distraction, capable of prolonged attention but occasionally distracted, vigilant

## 12.4 Concentration/Task Persistence:

Unable to maintain concentration for more than several minutes/duration of the examination, defective when compared with peers, preoccupations with self or other interfere with, by report able to maintain for several hours

It appeared that performance anxiety/fear of failure/fear of being found wanting/inadequate greatly interfered with his/her mental functioning, anxiety/preoccupations lessened/interfered with his/her concentration/immediate/recent memory

On SERIAL SEVENS : (<->)

Was able to subtract 7 from 100 (#) times/down to 2 accurately.

Did serial sevens down to (#) in (# seconds) with (#) errors when I stopped her/him.

Was able to do serial 7s (#) times before making an error

Self-corrected errors in the sequence.

Serial sevens were performed with (#) errors but subsequent subtractions were accurate based on the prior numbers.

Was un/able to subtract serial sevens accurately/could sustain concentration only to the first plateau/on (#) trials even with sincere effort.

Demonstrated adequate numerical reasoning but incorrect computations because of interfering anxiety

Shows decrements/lessening/limitations of mental efficiency

## 12.5 Memory:

INDICATIONS OF DEFECT: (<->)

Forgetful, "absent-minded", confused, uncertain/expresses doubts, befuddled, muddled, foggy, dreamy presentation, "spaced out", detached, vague, hesitant, guesses/estimates/approximates, Ganser's syndrome, confabulates, falsifies, perseverates, contaminations, diffusions

CAPABILITY:

Can only recognize, sluggish recall, recalls only with much prompting/cueing, reproduces with much difficulty/inaccuracy

AMNESIA:

Anteriograde (loss of experiences or materials learned since pathology/trauma), retrograde (loss of premorbid learning), Total Global Amnesia, ictus amnèsique, fugue, amnestic disorder, Korsakoff's syndrome

PARAMNESIA:

*Fausse reconnaissance,* retrospective falsification, confabulation, *dejà vu, dejà entendu, jamais vu,* hypermnesia, anomia, agnosia, propagnosia

IMPACT OF MEMORY DEFECT ON PATIENT: (<->)

No/poor/effective/maximal use of compensatory mechanisms/coping skills, constricts lifestyle, ignores, denies

SUMMARY STATEMENTS:

Un/able to recall three objects/words after five/ten minutes of different/unrelated activities
Faulty, limited recall, memory is limited/deficient/defective/a problem in all time frames

Un/able to give an account of his/her activities/life events in a chronological order
Memory, as reflected in his/her ability to provide an intact, sequential and logical history was
     defective/poor/adequate/normal/exceptional/unusual because ...
Memory for events in relationship to time was vague
Could not recall the time frames of school/work/family development/treatments
Client does not offer a rich description of important events from memory

Memory is organically intact but anxiety/depression interfere
Defective/normal/exceptional in processes of registration, retention and, recall
Defective/normal/exceptional in immediate/short-term retention/recent/recent past/remote memory.
Shows the pattern of memory deficits typical of those with/with a history of (diagnosis)
    ____ memory is not affected/normal but ____ memory is defective/exceptional
Remote and recent memories appear to be intact but there is an emptiness and lack of color in his/her
    descriptions of critical events

## 12.6 Information:

Limited education was apparent/demonstrated in low levels of the information typically acquired in
    grade school.
Considering his/her cultural background, level of formal and self-education her/his information was...
Impoverished/deficient fund of information/general knowledge, unaware of current/practical/general
    information, doesn't know the facts regarding his/her culture
His/her fund of factual knowledge is low/extensive/spotty
He/she is unaware of many basic factual, measurement, historical, and geographical concepts

## 12.7 Stream of Thought: (see also section 8.6 Speech as a Reflection of Cognition)

AMOUNT/PRODUCTIVITY: (<->)

| Impoverished | laconic | Normal | rapid | Flight of |
|---|---|---|---|---|
| paucity | moves slowly | spontaneous | overabundant | ideas |
| restricted | hesitant | average | "logorrhea" | |
| decreased | slowed | | copious | |
| unelaborated | | | | |
| under-productive | | | | |

# ABNORMAL Mental Status

CONTINUITY/COHERENCE: (<->) (see also section 8.6 Speech)

Word salad, incomprehensible, incoherent, chaotic, repetitive, perseverative

Neologisms, condensations, clang associations, loosened associations, thought/associational disturbance/disorder, cognitive slippage, blocked, over-inclusive, 'silly' conclusions

Tangential, drifting, circumstantial, derailment, rambling, discursive, digressive/digresses, circuitous, circular, "rattles on", irrelevant, distracted, no stepwise progressions, no logical sequences, lacking internal logic, connects associations by small and unusual similarities, needed to be refocussed/redirected

Goal-directed, clear cause-and-effect thinking, logical, coheres with questions asked, pertinent, sequential, relevant, coherent, to-the-point, rational, linear

PREOCCUPATIONS: (see also sections 13.3 Delusions and 13.13 Obsessions)

S/he is immersed in issues/themes of:

| | |
|---|---|
| Mental health | Religion |
| obsessions | over-piety |
| compulsions | excessive prayer |
| fears/phobias | blasphemous ideas |
| symptoms | denigrating activities |
| | irreligious practices/acts |
| Death and dying | fears/delusions about clergy/theology |
| suicide | |
| homicide | Relationships |
| dying | self-centeredness |
| morbid thoughts | guilt, sinfulness |
| losses | shame/embarrassment |
| | sexuality |

Somatic/hypochondriacal concerns
current physical illness, mortal illnesses, popular diseases
S/he is understandably and appropriately preoccupied with her/his health
His/her thoughts about ___ (e.g. health problems) dominate his/her thinking but are not exclusive or preoccupying.

Philosophy                                        His/her plight


THOUGHT DISTURBANCE:

See sections 12.8 Reasoning, and 8.6 Speech continuity



DISSOCIATION: (<->)

Day-dreaming, fanciful, trance, hysterical attack/episode, amnesia, fugue, somnambulism, automatic writing, out of body experience, extra-terrestrial travel, previous lives lived

OTHER:

| | | |
|---|---|---|
| Fails to answer questions | Loss of goal | Inter-penetration of themes |
| Over-inclusive | Loss of segmental set | |

## 12.8 Reasoning/Abstract Thinking/Concept Formation:
As assessed by means of similarities, absurdities, proverbs and concepts used in the evaluation

LEVEL OF INTERPRETATION:  (<->)

Greatly defective, failed to grasp nature of question, overly-concrete, personification, bizarreification, delusional, it was not possible to find proverbs simple enough for him/her to interpret

Concrete (noted only surface features or appearance aspects of stimuli), offers only very specific examples, paraphrases, reasons in a concrete manner, stimulus-bound associations, "I've heard that one before" (without elaboration)

Simplistic, difficulty with concept formation/judgment, similarities/differences, similarities/comparative analogies, absurdities, abstraction, proverbs

Couldn't use appropriate/expected levels of abstraction in dealing with test materials, mixes up categories in hierarchies, poor abstract thinking and concept-handling ability, degree of generalization was over-broad/narrow, some difficulty with reasoning at an easy/moderately difficult/difficult level

Functional levels of interpretation, responds only in terms of the uses for the stimulus item

Offered popular/unusual/idiosyncratic/antisocial interpretations

Abstracted common properties of the stimuli (noted relationships between stimuli/shared structural features) used principles, reasoned abstractly, offers similar proverbs/spontaneous re-phrasings, comprehensive level reasoning

Overly abstract, attended only to selected/irrelevant aspects of stimuli, artistic, philosophical, obscure, arcane references, highly theoretical, Byzantine

PRACTICAL REASONING: (See also 12.12 Judgement)

is defective requiring close support/monitoring to avoid loss/damage/exploitation, would be easily mislead and swindled/misused/taken advantage of
Was sufficient for independent living/assisting his/her supportive persons
Has substantial defects in his/her capacity to appreciate common/consensual reality
His/her thoughts are rational but not realistic

LOGICAL INFERENCE:

Faulty inductive/deductive inference/reasoning, reaches conclusions based on false/faulty premises, errors of logic and judgement, incorrect conclusions
Autistic, dereistic, idiosyncratic, *non-sequiturs, pars pro toto,* trance logic, paleologic

## 12.9 Arithmetic: (see also section 22.4 Math Ability)

OVERALL: (<->)

Anumerate, lacks practical/everyday/survival/basic mathematical skills, dyscalculia
His/her skills are approximately equivalent to those mastered in school grade __(#)

FINANCIAL: (see section 21.7 Financial)

## 12.10 Question Handling: (see also section 12.8 Stream of thought)

Did not understand give and take of question and answer format/did not grasp nature of questions, gave inappropriate responses, not relevant, nor logical, nor goal directed

## 12.11 Social Maturity: (see also 12.12 Social judgement)

When/as compared with others of same age/culture/education s/he demonstrated ....

IRRESPONSIBILITY: (see also sections 10.5 Guilt and 25.2 Antisocial personality)

Denies/lies about responsibilities, steals/destroys other's property, cheats, blames innocents, shows no guilt, offers no explanations, fakes guilt, offers only empty"phoney" apologies, not remorseful, falsely begs/pleads, "crocodile tears", refuses to pay debts/for property destroyed

On the job s/he resists/doesn't cooperate with/ignores/defies rules/directions/deadlines, starts many tasks but does not complete any, manipulates coworkers inot doing his/her work, needs close/continuous supervision, Absent WithOut Leave/slips away, tardy/takes too many/over-long rest periods/breaks/leaves early, intoxicated at work

SELF-CENTEREDNESS: (see also section 25.11 Narcissistic personality)

Calls others names/insults, manipulates, unrealistic/lacks/only immediate goals, selfish, uncaring, resents limits, self indulgent, impulsive, arousal seeking, acts out

FINANCIAL:

Doesn't manage funds well, squanders monies, impulsive/inappropriate/useless/wasteful purchases,

SOCIAL:

Resistant to authorities (parents, supervisor, police, human service professionals), chooses/imitates inappropriate or pathological models, touches others/without consent/self inappropriately

Has only limited contact with others so little opportunity to behave inappropriately
Teases, threatens vaguely/to leave/revenge/destruction of property/violence, threatens when confronted with own irresponsible behaviors, intimidates

## 12.12 Social/Moral Judgement and Knowledge: (see also sections 12.11 Social Maturity and 12.15 Decision Making)

POOR:

> Engaged in actions harmful to self
> Makes blatantly defective and self-damaging choices
> Has been taken advantage of repeatedly
> Not discriminating in choice of companions
> Heedless, reckless, feckless, careless
> Judgement is intact in terms of understanding (e.g. the demand characteristics of social settings) but
> > not in terms of behaviors
>
> Will make major decisions without sufficient information/impulsively/depending on hearsay/because
> > he/she doesn't want to refuse a friend, impulsive, immature, infantile, awkward, irresponsible
> Has impaired ability to make reasonable and realistic life decisions
> Seems guided by false beliefs
>
> Acted contrary to acceptable behavior
> Did not comprehend the expected/usual consequences of his/her behaviors nor the impact/impression
> > made upon others
> Inadequately cognizant/aware of the basic social conventions
> Has difficulty with performing the tasks supportive of/related to carrying out the decisions made
> Given the defective quality of her/his thinking/understanding judgement has to be impaired
> Has a lifelong history of ineffective coping

GOOD: (<->)

Responsible, understood/anticipates the likely consequences of his/her behavior/actions, distinguishes socially acceptable behaviors from those not and acts on this understanding, learns from other's mistakes/vicariously/ or from correction/instruction

> Has common sense, had reasonable responses to hypothetical judgement questions, sought treatment
> for medical/psychological problems, can plan ahead, learns from experience/mistakes/feedback/
> "street-smart"
>
> > Able to identify and control behaviors which would be harmful to her/him and contrary to
> > acceptable rules/beyond the limits of the society/social group/community, learns from other's
> > mistakes/vicariously/instruction

## 12.13 Test Judgement:
Evaluation of subject's judgement as based on a comparison with premorbid state or expected ability based on intellect/age/education/social experience is ...

> Performance on the judgement questions asked/tests used was poor/adequate/good/normal/expected/
> > excellent which suggests that in the external/social/'real' world s/he would ...

## 12.14 Motivation for Change: (see also section 16. Prognosis)

Moitivation is limited by low frustration tolerance, dependency, ambivalence, low initiative
Motivation is needed for change/therapy/habilitation/rehabilitation/self-improvement

## Affect:  See section 10. Emotional/Affective Symptoms

## 12.15 Decision Making: (see also section 12.12 Social/Moral Judgement.) (<->)

Easily confused, easily overwhelmed in choice situations, lacks understanding of options, fails to evaluate choices

Indecisive, flounders, dithers, procrastinates, ponders endlessly, avoids decision situations, reverses decisions, wishy-washy, vacillates

Unable to carry out choices verbalized, deficient in carrying out instructions/in finishing tasks started, can make only simple/work related decisions

Decisive, effective, follows through, tolerates frustration/ambiguity/delay/errors/peers/ setbacks/changes/ambivalence

## 12.16 Learning:

Does not learn new information/material with repeated exposures

Easily grasps concepts and methods on first trial, generalizes from earlier situations, uses theoretical models, alters own behaviors in light of experience/changed situation/requests from others

Curious, attentive

## 12.17 Other/Summary Statements for an ABNORMAL Mental Status:

Impaired mental control functions
Unable to shift cognitive sets, rigid, inflexible
Defective sequencing ability
Ranchos Los Amigos cognitive functioning level of __ (I to VIII)
Presence of a dementing process
Considering client's age and education....
Based on interview behavior, I believe ....
Has only fleeting contact with "reality"

**For a Child**
Soft neurological signs (incoordination, poor balance, poor speech, delayed development, etc.), Funny Looking Kid,

# 13. Standard Statements for ABNORMAL Signs, Symptoms and Syndromes of Disorder

This list of signs and symptoms EXCLUDES all those referring to COGNITIVE MENTAL FUNCTIONING. (For those, see section 12. Abnormal Mental Status)

The categories of statements are presented here in alphabetical order as no hierarchy is agreed upon.

Note: Remember to report positive as well as negative findings.

## 13.1 Attention Deficit Disorder

A primary difficulty maintaining a focus of attention against distraction and which results in the disorganization of behavior as seen in inattention, impulsivity or hyperactivity.

BEHAVIOR:

Fidgets, wriggles, twists, squirms, does not sit through an interview or meal, always "on the go", prefers to run rather than walk, climbs on furniture, hops/skips/jumps rather than walking, fiddles with objects, taps/hits and makes noises, moves unnecessarily, disrupts shopping and family visits, acts 'wild' in crowded settings, babysitters complain about his/her behavior

Shifts from one incomplete task to another, does not finish what he/she starts, rushes/jumps from one topic of conversation to another, does not complete assignments on time, starts work before receiving instructions

Non-compliant, does not comply with instructions, does not sit when told to, defiant, resistant, "sasses"/"talks back", argumentative, oppositional, breaks school/game's rules, unable to follow a routine

Does not play quietly, talks excessively, does everything in the noisiest way

Needs constant/continual/one-to-one supervision/monitoring/teaching, needs closeness and eye-contact to understand instructions

Adapts to changes in situation/routine/personnel poorly

Poor fine motor skills, is disorganized with possessions

Impulsive, reacts without considering

Senseless, repetitive, eccentric behaviors

COGNITIVE:

Easily distracted, lessened ability to sustain attention/concentration on school task/work/play
Needs/asks for repetitions of instructions, gets confused, doesn't "listen" although s/he hears normally, inattentive to significant details
Has low self-esteem/image, feels worthless
Low concern for accuracy, neatness or quality of work, disregards instructions
Ignores consequences of own behaviors

**Abn. Sx.**

> .*Academic difficulties with:* counting, time-telling, recognizing letters, word finding, stops in middle of a sentence or thought, confuses/reverses word order in sentences, mistakes similar sounding words, adds/substitutes/reverses letters/words/sounds, copies letters and words poorly
> Low short-term memory skills, fails to remember sequences, loses place when reading
> Disorganized work habits: does not study/prepare, organize, protect own work, do problem's steps in sequence

## AFFECT:

> Unpredictable and unrelated mood changes, often depressed/blue/sad, pessimistic, gloomy
> His/her feelings are easily hurt, cries very easily
> Easily angered/upset, gets overexcited

## SOCIAL:

> Interrupts/intrudes/"butts in", talks out in class, shouts out answers or comments, makes disruptive noises, does not wait his/her turn in group situations, no patience, impulsive, excitable, explosive
> Fights with sibs/peers/teachers, violent, aggressive, destructive, plays "tough guy", often involved in physically dangerous activities, hits/punches/strikes/kicks/bites, cries/withdraws, verbal conflict/insults/harasses/teases/coerces/intimidates/manipulates/"bosses"/provokes, disrupts other children's activities, betrays friends, peers avoid/reject him/her

## CONDUCT DISORDER - SOCIALIZED

> Selfishly accepts without any desire to return favors
> Makes an effort on a task or toward others only if it serves his/her interests
> Believes others are against him/he is being treated unfairly
> Will cheat in order to win, eill lie to be seen as the winner
> Stubbornly resists other's ways of doing things

## CONDUCT DISORDER - AGGRESSIVE

> Aggressive, violent, dangerous, assaults, fights with anyone, threatens (see Social, above)
> Lies/cheats/breaks any rules/steals/denies truth/blames others
> Swears offensively, vulgarisms

---

## 13.2 Compulsions: (see also section 13.13 Obsessions)
Repetitive, "purposeful" behaviors performed according to rules. The actions are resisted yet performed, and are tension-relieving.

S engages in *rituals* for meals, sleep, dressing, house cleaning, washing, defecation, school/work tasks, etc.

S feels compelled to repeatedly *check* the house, kitchen, windows and doors, dangerous objects, children, etc.

S feels compelled to repeatedly *touch, count, arrange and rearrange* objects

Other: kleptomania, trichotilomania, "nymphomania", "satyriasis"

Client denied problems with common compulsions

## 13.3 Delusions:
Non-reality based beliefs, essentially unshakeable, defended despite evidence, and unique to the individual or not supported by culture or subculture.

DEGREE: (<->)

Faint suspiciousness, distrust, magical thinking, personalized meanings, overvalued ideas, ideas of reference, allusions to trickery and deceit, believes in ... but this in not of delusional force, convinced of truth of, formed delusions/deluded, pseudologica fantastica, organized/well organized/systematized and extensive system of beliefs, lives in a fantasy world   The

delusions

are fixed/trusted/doubted/rejected/denied.
are extensive/circumscribed/isolated/encapsulated.
show a high/low/fragmented degree of organization.
are shared with others/family members (*folie à deux* or *à trois*).
rarely/often/continually expressed
elicited easily/with difficulty/only with exceptionally trusted others

CONTENTS of the delusion are of:

| Grandiosity | persecution | religion | nihilistic | suicide | disease |
|---|---|---|---|---|---|
| | reference | | poverty | homicide | somatic |
| omniscience | following | fantasies | fears | approaching | hypochondriacal |
| omnipotence | influence | wishes | | death | phobic |
| extraordinary | alien control | erotomania | | | distorted body |
| abilities | misidentif- | sexual identity | | self-deprecation | image |
| | ication | | | self-accusation | |
| | | obsessions | | guilt | zooanthropic |
| | | preoccupations | | derogation | |
| | infidelity | monomanical focus | | shame | |
| | jealousy | worries | | sin | |

Other: having neglected an urgent responsibility, caused harm to befall another person, inadvertently contaminated others, sexual identity, self-referential ideas, being followed, people making fun of her/him, trying to control her, people know his thoughts

The *effects* of the delusions on the subject's life situation seems to be large/limiting/minor/circumscribed.

The *origin* of the delusions seems to have been in ___ .

FIRST-RANK or SCHNEIDERIAN DELUSIONS:

Primary delusional perception
Delusional elaboration of a percept
Passive reception of a somatic sensation
Thought transmission/broadcasting/insertion/withdrawal
Clouding
'Made' impulses/volitional acts/feelings
Voices arguing with the subject in the third person
Voices making a continuous commentary on the subject's actions
Voices speaking the subject's thoughts aloud (écho de pensées)

SECOND-RANK DELUSIONS: These are delusions based on or about other psychological phenomena such as hallucinations, other delusions, or on affects such as mania.

## 13.4 Depersonalization and Derealization: Loss of the continuity of consciousness, identity and motor behaviors.

Reports observing oneself from a distance/corner of the room, as if outside one's body, body appears altered, feels mechanical/robot-like

Self-estrangement, extreme feelings of unreality/detachment from self/environment/surroundings, "dreaming"/living a dream, as if the world were not real

Experienced her thoughts as not her own, as if his body and mind were not linked

## 13.5 Depression - (see section 10.4 Depression and 5.25 Suicide)

## 13.6 Eating disorders:

ANOREXIA NERVOSA:

> Cachexia/cachetic, emaciated, amenorrhea, bradycardia, hypothermia, edema, laxative/diuretic misuse/abuse, fasting, starvation, over-exercising, distorted body image so believes s/he is always too fat, "food phobia"

BULIMIA:

> Bulimarexia (not a widely accepted term), bulimia nervosa, gorging, binge eating, self-induced vomiting/emesis, binge-purge cycling, gastric dilation

OBESITY: (see also section 8.2 Behavioral observations, weight)

> Factitious, obsessional concerns, overweight, obese, chronic, stable, compulsive dieting, escalating weight over diets

PICA

## 13.7 Intermittent-Explosive Disorder: (See section 13.11 Impulse control)

## 13.8 Extra-Pyramidal Symptoms:

Involuntary muscle movements: lip smacking, tongue rolling, tongue thrusting, jaw clenching, drooling, mask-like facies, woodenness, rigidity, cogwheel rigidity, tics, tremors, dyskinesias, tardive dyskinesia, oculo-gyric crises, torsion spasms, internal tension

> Blurred vision, dry mouth, slowing, restlessness, excessive sedation/oversleeping/sleepiness

## 13.9 Hallucinations:

SENSORY MODALITY: EXAMPLES

| | |
|---|---|
| Visual: | Unformed/lights/flashes, formed/people/animals/things, Lilliputian |
| Tactile (haptic): | Electricity, sexual sensations, tickling |
| Kinesthetic: | Creeping, crawling, biting, gnawing, twisting, churning, pains |
| Auditory: | Noises or voices (see below) |
| Olfactory: | Disgusting/repulsive/objectionable odors, of death or disease |
| Gustatory: | Poisons, acid, foul tastes |
| Visceral/somatic: | Phantom Limb, "hollow insides", "rotting insides" |
| Vestibular: | Sensations of flying, falling, lightness |
| Synesthesia: | e.g.. smells red |

CONTENTS OF AUDITORY HALLUCINATIONS::

Noises: whistling, ringing
Voices: whose?, male or female, age
Disconnected words, muffled voices, his/her own thoughts, remarks addressed to him/her,
      informative, friendly, benign, comforting, helpful, socially focused, arguing, commenting,
      grandiose, malevolent, accusatory, berating, persecutory, harassing, hateful, spiteful,
      threatening, controlling, compelling, premonitory, hortatory/imperative/commanding,
      isolating
Idiosyncratic themes

ATTITUDE TOWARD HALLUCINATIONS: (<->)

Ego-alien, frightened, terrified, resisted/struggled against, engages in conversations/dialogue with
      imaginary interlocutor, comforting, ego-syntonic, accepted

(<->) Convinced of their reality, vivid fantasy, "altered state", impossibility, "only a
      fantasy", doubting its reality/own perceptions, making various efforts to control/cope with it,
      "bizarre", "rare"

CIRCUMSTANCES OF OCCURRENCE:

Hypnogogic, hypnopompic, with delirium, in withdrawal, flashbacks, spontaneously, unbidden,
extent of cultural/situational anxiety/external stimuli on the hallucinatory experience,
undiscoverable relationship to circumstances

INTERPERSONAL ASPECTS:

Hallucinations are denied by the patient but s/he seems to be responding to internal stimuli
They involve small/moderate/great distortion of consensual reality

OTHER HALLUCINATIONS:

Of presence of another person, extracampine, autoscopy, *doppelgänger*, replacement of another/self

## 13.10 Illusions: (see also section 5.13 Illusions)

Sense deceptions, deceptive sensations, visual/auditory/tactile distortions, speeded up or slowed
      passage of time
Macropsia, micropsia, Lilliputian, gigantism

YVONNE DAVIS

## 13.11 Impulse Control/ViolenceAggression: (see section 10.2 Anger)

TYPES OF IMPULSES:

Hostile, aggressive, violent, destructive, amorous, sexual

DEGREE OF CONTROL: (<->)

| Patient | Volatile | Impulsive | Violent |
|---|---|---|---|
| tolerant | looses temper | may attack | explosive |
| inhibited | easily irritated | short fuse | "blows his/her top" |
| thoughtful | low frustration | impetuous | combative |
| deliberate | tolerance | hot headed | assaultive |
| controlled | quicksilver | flares up | aggressive |
| over-cautious | rash | quick tempered | lashes out |
| staid | leaves situation | "flies off the handle" | belligerent |
| | stormy | abrupt | |
| cool-headed | hasty | precipitous | |
| restrained | easily offended | unpredictable | |
| self-possessed | excitable | incontinent | |
| | irritable | reckless | |
| | | outbursts | |

FEARS HE/SHE MAY:

Embarrass him/herself, lose control, "wet pants"/lose bladder control, faint
Harm self or others, homicidal ideation, threats, behavior
Not be able to resist impulses to commit delinquent of illegal acts

REASON'S INFLUENCE:

Acts without weighing alternatives, likely to act without consideration of alternatives/with little hesitation, unreflective, acts without examination, unmediated, "acts on spur of the moment", easily agitated, off-handed/ill-considered actions, self-centered actions, seeks immediate gratification of urges, heedless, willful, limited intellectual control over expression of impulses, poor planning

VIOLENCE AGAINST:

Objects/property/self/family/strangers/women/animals/authority figures/weaker persons, any available target, outside the home

ANTISOCIAL BEHAVIOR:

Obstructiveness, cheating, lying, stealing, crimes, arrests, fighting, forceful aggression, irresponsibility

CORRELATES OF SERIOUS AGGRESSION:

| | |
|---|---|
| Tortures animals | Profitless damaging of property, especially one's own |
| Hidden aggressive acts | Apparently purposeless aggressive actions |
| Fighting with weaker opponents | Careless of risk of self harm when acting aggressively |
| Pride in history of aggression | "Out of control" when aggressive |
| Stealing, lying | Plans aggressive actions |

## 13.12 Insight: (<->)

NIL OR LITTLE:

> No insight, blindly uncritical of own behavior, denies illness/symptoms, aware of problem but blames others/circumstances/physical factors/something unknown or mysterious for problems, rebuts psychological or motivational interpretations of his behavior, fights the system and does little or nothing to help her/himself, fatalistic resignation

> Superficial, shallow, platitudinous, difficulty in acknowledging the presence of psychological problems, self-deceiving, unable to focus on issues

> Denies, despite the evidence, that his/her current symptoms are important or that s/he needs help, or that he/she needs to change his/her attitude/behavior/feelings in some specific way, staff evaluations/findings were minimized, denied, obfuscated, and evaded in discussions with patient

SOME:

> Unable to make use of correct insights, only flashes of insight

> Continues trying to make sense of his/her psychotic thinking

FULL: (<->)

Believes he/she is ill, recognizes need for treatment, came to treatment voluntarily, labels own illness, takes medicines, attends therapy sessions, works in therapy, acknowledges psychological/physical/historical limitations present

> Accepts that his/her symptoms/problematic behaviors/failures in adaptation are at least in part due to his/her irrational thought/feelings/internal states, can identify the emotional/cognitive antecedents and consequents of symptomatic behaviors, recognizes relation of symptomatic behavior to (e.g. alcohol abuse) to emotional states, or to impact on life's duration/quality/satisfaction

>> Open to new ideas/perspectives on him/herself and other important people, self-aware, psychologically minded, accepts explanations offered by care-givers

>>> Understands outcomes of his behavior and is influenced by this awareness, is able to identify/distinguish/comprehend behaviors which would be contrary to social values/socially non-acceptable or personally counterproductive

>>> Can apply understanding to change actions/direction of his/her life, understands causes/dynamics/treatments/implications of his/her illness

---

Mood: General aspects of mood and descriptive terms for Anxiety, Depression, and Anger can be found in section 10.

## 13.13 Obsessions:
Involuntary, ego-dystonic, senseless/repugnant, intrusive thoughts or images which cannot be ignored or suppressed.

RUMINATIONS/REPETITIVE:

> Thoughts, music, names, titles, numbers, phrases, memories, images, impulses, religious ideas, etc.

> Monomania, monothematic thought trains, repetitive themes, erotomania, egomania, megalomania, overvalued ideas (e.g. dysmorphobia)

PREOCCUPATIONS: (see sections 12.7 Stream of thought and 13.3 Delusions)

## 13.14 Degree of Paranoia: (see also section 13.3 Delusions)

DEGREE: (<->)

Persecutory ideas, demonstrations of suspiciousness, distrust, paranoid trends, paranoid cognitive style, reported paranoid ideation, belief that everything is not as it should be, inappropriate suspiciousness

> Pervasive suspiciousness about everyone/everyone's actions, partially supported delusions, likely story of persecution, evidence of persecution, on guard, hyperalert, vigilant, spied on, plotted against, attempts made to to harm, attacks, attacks foiled

>> Systematized delusions, reinforced delusions

>>> Believes him/herself to be exceedingly virtuous, denies that he/she distrusts others, persistently naive about other's motives, believes him/herself to be especially sensitive, overvalues own subjective knowledge

## 13.15 Phobias:
Persistent, recognzed-as-unrealistic fears, high levels of circumscribed anxiety, and avoidance of the anxiety-arousing situations/animals/social settings/persons.

TYPES:

> Traumatically learned phobia, simple phobia, animal phobias, school phobia, social phobia, agoraphobia, acrophobia, algophobia, claustrophobia, xenophobia, zoophobia

Schneiderian symptoms: see section 13.3 Delusions

## 13.16 Sleep Disturbances: (see section 5.22 Sleep, for questions)
Avoid the use of the term insomnia alone as it has multiple meanings and so is vague.

> Difficulty Falling Asleep, initial insomnia
> Sleep Continuity Disturbance, interrupted/broken/fragmented sleep
> Early Morning Awakening, terminal insomnia
> Vivid Dreams (all but real, well organized contents, of neutral mood, felt as very different from usual dreaming, concerning persons and events from subject's remote past)
> Night Terrors (reported by other and not recalled by subject, sudden screaming, thrashing, or calling out, sleep is not interrupted or if awakened s/he cannot recall scream or reason for scream, whole episode not recalled in morning)
> Nightmares (frightening, often paranoid quality, recalled in morning and disruptive of sleep)
> Nocturnal vocalizations, nocturnal jerking/myoclonus, somnambulism (sleepwalking), apnea
> Narcolepsy, sleep paralysis, cataplexy, hypnogogic/hypnopompic hallucinations

OTHER:

> Total sleep time is decreased/increased/unaffected/normal/not determinable, asomnia, hyposomnia, hypersomnia, reversal of day/night cycle, "Lark" (morning alertness) or "Owl" (evening alertness with morning ineffectiveness)

## 13.17 Stress Tolerance: (see also section 24.3 Coping ability)

Low/moderate/high, frustration tolerance, ability to delay gratifications, tolerance for ambiguity/uncertainty/ conflict/low information/structure, hardiness

## 13.18 Substance Abuse: (See also section 5.23 Substance Abuse Questions) (<->)

Showed signs of intoxication: smell of alcohol on breath, slurred speech, lessened concentration, slowed movements and responses, loosened associations, flat or exaggerated affect expression, disoriented, dozed off, defective memory, discoordination, unusual pupil size

IDENTIFICATION AS AN ADDICT: (<->)

Does not agree to any intemperate use/drinking problem/bingeing/alcoholism, brags about sprees, admits to intemperate use of alcohol/drugs, "Not addicted", addicted only to one of several drugs used, acknowledges the negative consequences of his/her use but fails to recognize using as self-defeating, verbally identifies as an addict but shows no changed behaviors such as improved social skills, resisting/avoiding high temptation situations, or alternative problem solutions which would support freedom from addiction, too easily admits his/her alcoholism, identifies self as "an alcoholic", demonstrates insightful identification as an addict/cross addict through change in identification, lifestyle, relationships, and behaviors

Concerning her insight, she treats her alcoholism with indifference and resignation, and feels hopeless and defeated so that she continues to abuse alcohol as a lifestyle

S/he rationalized about her/his drinking in an illogical manner suggesting its value to her/him. For example, s/he uses it to sleep, control the 'shakes', loosen up, and reports that being drunk saved her/his life in an auto accident.

MOTIVATION FOR RECOVERY (<->)

Hopeless of change, self-medicates with (substances), seeks only to avoid problems from addiction/use, or to please other people and no to change own symptomatic behaviors, verbalizes motivation but seems insincere, reports hope, demonstrates hope through new behaviors

AA AND OTHER TREATMENTS:

Client denies need for/denigrates/rejects/attends grudgingly/mechanically/regularly/daily/ is proud of membership in AA, client knows name of/is a Sponsor

S/he attended rehabilitation programs with only short-term/time limited/progressively greater/excellent success at abstinence/control

History of previous chemical dependency treatments, duration, longest period of sobriety afterward

**13.19 Suicide:** (See also sections 10.4 for suicide as an emotional component of depression and 5.25 for questions about suicidal ideation)

DEGREE OF SUICIDAL IDEATION AND BEHAVIOR: (<->)

"Impossible", highly unlikely, improbable, against strongly held religious beliefs or philosophy of life, "never" considered, wishes to live, reasons for living exceed reasons for dying

Passive death wishes or ideas, subintended suicide

Considered and abandoned, flimsy rationales for refusing suicide, unlikely, not currently considered, fleeting thoughts of suicide, passive suicide attempt, would leave death to chance, would avoid steps necessary to save or maintain life

Thoughts/ideation, wishes to end life, expressed ambivalence, inclination, wonders if s/he will make it through this, raises questions of life after death,

Verbalizations, recollections of other's suicide, plans, discusses methods and means, stated intent, used as a threat, thoughts of self-mutilation, asks others to help kill him/her

Behaviors, gesture, non/low lethality, non-dangerous method, acts of self-mutilation, symbolic/ineffective/harmless attempts, parasuicide, command hallucinations with suicidal intent, wishes without plan

Attempt(s), deliberateness, action planning, method/means selected/acquired, high lethality method, giving away possessions, arranging affairs, wrote note, told others of intent

Persistent/continuous/continual efforts, unrelenting preoccupation

INCREASED RISK OF SUICIDE IS GENERALLY RELATED TO:

Hopelessness, pessimism, acceptance of unalterability of painful situation, finality, irresolvable, incurable, permanent

Caucasian (3X more adult and 2X more adolescent succeeders than Blacks and other minorities)[1]
Male (3X more succeeders, 1/3 as many attempters than females)
Medical, dental and mental health professionals, lawyers, etc.
Young adult or geriatric,
Most succeeders are white, US-born men aged 45-60

Somatic/vegetative aspects of depression
Refused to accept help now
Highly dependent personality
Serious medical illness or disability
Increased irritation
Currently intoxicated, or long history of alcohol abuse without current drinking

Confusion and disorganization of thoughts
Extreme anxiety or panics
Prior inpatient psychiatric treatment

Recent angry, enraged or violent behavior

Multiple attempts (half of succeeders have one previous attempt)
Clearly determinable time of suicide attempt
High lethality of past attempts or current plan
Attempts with little chance of discovery

Recent attempts
Attempts on anniversaries of significant events

---

[1]I am grateful to Robert W. Moffie, Ph.D for correction and clarification of this issue.

**Abn. Sx.**

Failure to perform major life role behavior
Self evaluation is excessively based upon performance in standard gender roles

Divorced status, repeated, or in last 6 months    Never-married or widowed status

Living alone
Living with other than family members    Partner is also suicidal
Few or no family members available    Family history of death by suicide

No friends nearby    No warm, close interdependent relationships

Refusal or inability to cooperate with treatment

Considering homicide as well as suicide    History of criminal behavior

Note: You may also need to inquire about homicide or violence (See section 13.11)

---

## Thought's Continuity, Content and other aspects: (see section 8.5 Speech as a Reflection of Cognition)

# Conversions of Scores Based on the Normal Curve of Distibution

| Percentage of cases under portions of the normal curve | | 0.13 | | 2.14 | | 13.59 | | 34.13 | | 34.13 | | 13.59 | | 2.14 | | 0.13 | |

| Standard Deviations -SD or σ | -4 | | -3 | | -2 | | -1 | | 0 | | +1 | | +2 | | +3 | | +4 |

| Cumulative percentages | | | 0.1 | | 2.3 | | 15.9 | | 50.0 | | 84.1 | | 97.7 | | 99.9 | | | |

| Percentile equivalents | | | 1 | 5 | 10 | 20 | 30 40 50 60 | 70 | 80 | 90 | 95 | 99 | | | |

| Stanines (Mean = 5, SD = 2) | | | 1 | 2 | 3 | 4 | 5 | 6 | 7 | 8 | 9 | | | |
| Percent in each Stanine | | | 4 | 7 | 12 | 17 | 20 | 17 | 12 | 7 | 2 | | | |

| Z - Scores (Mean = 0, SD = 1) | -4.0 | -3.0 | -2.0 | -1.0 | 0.0 | +1.0 | +2.0 | +3.0 | +4.0 |

| T - Scores (Mean = 50, SD = 10) | | 20 | 30 | 40 | 50 | 60 | 70 | 80 | |

| Deviation IQs (Mean = 100, SD = 15) | 40 | 55 | 70 | 85 | 100 | 115 | 130 | 145 | |

| Wechsler Subtest Scaled Scores (Mean = 10, SD = 3) | 1 | 4 | 7 | 10 | 13 | 16 | 19 | |

| Binet IQs (Mean = 100, SD = 16) | 50 | 66 | 84 | 100 | 116 | 132 | 148 | |

# 14. Diagnosis/Impression

## 14.1 Summary of Positive Findings:

Signs, symptoms, syndromes, patterns (See section 13. for Abnormal Signs and Symptoms)

## 14.2 Diagnosis is Qualified as:

Initial, deferred, principal, additional/co-morbidity, rule out ..., admitting, tentative, working, final, discharge, in remission, quiescent

DSM-III-R offers specification as: Mild, Moderate, Severe, In Partial Remission, Residual State, or Full Remission

## 14.3 DSM III-R* (This section is modified, except as indicated, from the Diagnostic and Statistical Manual, version three, revised, of the American Psychiatric Association, 1987).

AXIS 1 - All Disorders (maladaptive patterns or clinical syndromes) except Personality Disorders and Specific Developmental Disorders

AXIS 2 - Personality Disorders (long standing, in adults) and Specific Developmental Disorders (in children)

AXIS 3 - Physical Disorders and other conditions present

AXIS 4 - Severity of Psychosocial Stressors:
Consider the last year's time period, assume an "average" person of the same sociocultural values, and number of stressors

*Consider the following categories of stressors: (From DSM III and III-R):*

| | |
|---|---|
| Health (illness, injury, disability) | Work, occupational situations |
| Bereavement | School |
| Love and marriage, conjugal relations | Financial |
| Parenting | Legal |
| Family stressors (for children and adolescents) | Developmental |
| Other familial (extended family) relationships | Psychosocial |
| Housing/environmental, living circumstances | Miscellaneous |
| Other relationships (voluntary, friendships) outside the family, interpersonal | |

---

* The DSM-III-R is available from American Psychiatric Press, Inc., Order Department, 1400 K Street, N.W. Washington, D.C. 20005 or 1-800-368-5777 for (as of 1989) $39.95 (hardcover, Item # 42-01801) or $29.95 (paperback, Item # 42-019-X) plus $3.00 shipping and handling.

## Diagnosis

ADULT'S NUMERICAL RATING AND EXAMPLES: [Stressors may be acute (less than 6 months) or enduring.]

1 - None - No apparent relevant psychosocial stressors or enduring circumstances
2 - Mild - e.g. Broke up with boyfriend/girlfriend, child left home, started or graduated from school, family arguments or job dissatisfaction, residence in high-crime neighborhood
3 - Moderate - e.g. Marriage or marital separation, loss of job, marital discord or serious financial problems, single parenthood
4 - Severe - e.g. Divorce or birth of first child, unemployment or poverty
5 - Extreme - e.g. Death of a spouse, serious physical illness diagnosed, victim of rape, ongoing sexual or physical abuse, serious chronic illness in self or child
6 - Catastrophic - e.g. Multiple family deaths, death of a child, suicide of spouse, hostage or concentration camp experience, war, natural disaster
0 - Unspecified. - Inadequate information or no change in condition

CHILD OR ADOLESCENT'S NUMERICAL RATING: (Stressors may be acute or enduring)

1 - None - No apparent relevant psychosocial stressors or enduring circumstances
2 - Mild - e.g. Broke up with boyfriend/girlfriend, change in school, family arguments or overcrowded living quarters
3 - Moderate - e.g. Expelled from school, birth of a sibling, chronic parental discord or disabling illness in parent
4- Severe - e.g. Divorce of parents, harsh or rejecting parents, multiple foster home placements, arrest, chronic life-threatening illness in parent, unwanted pregnancy
5 - Extreme - e.g. Death of a parent, severe or recurrent sexual or physical abuse
6 - Catastrophic - e.g. Death of both parents, chronic life-threatening illness
0 - Unspecified. - Inadequate information or no change in condition

AXIS 5 - Global Assessment of Functioning (This is an abbreviated version and does not list examples) Ratings are made of current level of psychological/social/physical functioning and for highest level in past year .

ADULT'S NUMERICAL RATING: (Use intermediate numbers where appropriate, e.g 45, 68)

| | |
|---|---|
| 90 - 81 | Good in all areas - e.g. Social, occupational (or school) and psychological functioning is without notable problems. Symptoms are absent or minimal. |
| 80 - 71 | Only slight impairment - e.g. Temporary inefficiency in occupation or schoolwork. Symptoms, if present, are temporary and expectable/normal for stressors. |
| 70 - 61 | Some difficulty - e.g. In spite of overall functioning, person has some difficulties in social, occupational or school sphere. Retains some meaningful interpersonal relationships. If present, symptoms are mild. |
| 60 - 51 | Moderate difficulty - e.g. Moderate disruption of social, occupational or school functioning *or* symptoms of moderate severity, such as occasional panic attacks. |
| 50 - 41 | Serious difficulty - e.g. Any serious impairment in social, occupational or school functioning *or* serious symptoms such as suicidal ideation or compulsive rituals. |
| 40 - 31 | Major impairments - e.g. Major impairment in several areas such as work, school, family relations, judgement, thinking, or mood, *or* shows some impairment of reality testing or communication. |

30 - 21    Unable to function - e.g. Inability to manage almost all areas of behavior considerably influenced by delusions, hallucinations, *or* seriously impaired judgement or communication

20 - 11    Some danger of hurting self or others - e.g. Some failure to maintain minimal standards of personal hygiene, *or* gross impairment in communication or judgement

10 - 1     Persistent danger - e.g. Person is judged to be a persistent danger to self or others *or* inability to maintain minimal standards of hygiene, *or* recent serious suicidal act having clear expectation of death

## CHILD NUMERICAL RATING:

91-100    Superior functioning in areas such as school, home and with peers, many interests and activities (groups, extracurricular, hobbies), likeable and confident, no symptoms or symptomatic level behaviors

81-90     Good overall functioning, secure but with possible transient difficulties and sometimes excessive "ordinary" worries such as exam anxiety, blowups with siblings

71-80     No more than slight impairment and some brief disturbance of behavior under life stresses such as parental separation, birth of a sib. Not considered deviant or distressing to others

61-70     Some difficulty in one area of functioning such as skipping school, petty theft, brief "bad moods", or self-doubts, poor schoolwork. Not seen as deviant by those who know child but others may express some concern

51-60     Sporadic difficulties in several areas. Disturbance seen only in dysfunctional settings

41-50     Moderately poor functioning in most areas or severe impairment in one area such as suicidal ideations, school refusal, rituals, conversion symptoms, anxiety attacks, aggressive episodes

31-40     Major impairment in several areas such as persistent aggression, isolating self, lethal suicide attempts, may require special schooling

21-30     Unable to function in almost all areas with severe limitations of communication or reality testing, and isolation

11-20     Requires close supervision to prevent self or other damage or to maintain personal hygiene or to manage severe communication deficits

0-10      Requires constant care and supervision due to deficits

# V CODES:

Consider the noting of these "conditions not attributable to a mental disorder that are a focus of attention or treatment."

---

**14.4 ICD-9-CM\*** (<u>I</u>nternational <u>C</u>lassification of <u>D</u>iseases, <u>9</u>th Edition, <u>C</u>linical <u>M</u>odification.) Compiled by the World Health Organization of the United Nations. It went into effect January 1, 1979.

A discussion of this manual and its mental disorders section with the code numbers and glossary definitions and clarifications are reprinted in the DSM-III-R book.

---

**14.5 CPT-4†** (Physician's Current Procedural Terminology, Fourth Edition) 1986, American Medical Association

---

**14.6 PTM§** (Procedure Terminology Manual) of Blue Cross/Blue Shield

---

## 14.7 Psychodynamic Treatment Evaluations:

Dynamic: psychosexual developmental levels, areas of conflict, mechanisms of defense/adaptation, character/personality structure, estimate of treatability, transference issues, ego strength, potential for acting out, identity, object relationships

---

## 14.8 Developmental Diagnosis:

Areas of developmental delays/normal functioning/advance

---

## 14.9 Strengths to Build Upon:

Vigor, drive, spirit, courage, determination, valor

Assets, resources, qualifications, reserves, possessions, skills, abilities, aptitudes, capabilities, knowledges, dexterity, talents, prowesses, proficiencies, competencies, experience, expertise

---

\* The ICD-9-CM is available from: CPHA Telemarketing, 1968 Green Road/P.O. Box 1809, Ann Arbor MI 48106-1809, Phone (303) 769-6511 X 4424 or 4552

† The CPT-4 is available from: Book and Pamphlet Fulfillment, American Medical Association, P.O. Box 10946, Chicago, IL 60610-09436

§ The PTM is available from your local Blue Cross-Blue Shield Organization

# 15. Recommendations

## 15.1 Treatment Recommendations/Disposition:

Treatability estimate

Continue current treatment(s), additional/concurrent treatments referral, hospital/program/therapist transfer, discharge

Change diet to ...
Change exercise to ...
Change social/recreational etc activities to ..., increase activities outside the home/family, take on volunteer activities such as ...
Bibliotherapy assignments such as ...

Further evaluations/diagnostic studies: physical/medical, intellectual, personality, neuropsychological, custody, family, audiological, speech/language, occupational/vocational, educational/academic

Medication)s)s: (name(s)) at a starting dosage of ... for a duration of .... with instructions regarding ... to be supervised/administered by patient/family/clinic staff/school nurse/Visiting Nurse

Counseling or psychotherapy: with whom, where, frequency, duration, mode/format, technique(s).

Behavior referral: self-control training, Anger Management, parenting skills/child management training, Parent Effectiveness Training

Other therapies: expressive therapies (art, music, dance/movement, poetry), crisis intervention only, staff monitoring, bibliotherapy, assertiveness training, spousal/family support, Aftercare services, consciousness raising, sex therapy, marital counseling

Specialized community support groups: grief counseling, victim support services, Mothers Against Drunk Driving, Parents of Murdered Children, Candlelighters, Reach for Recovery, Parents Anonymous, Recovery groups, Take Off Pounds Sensibly,

12 Step programs for many addictive behaviors: Narcotics, Alcohol, Overeaters, Gamblers Anonymous

Educational groups: Toastmasters International, Marriage Encounter, local college/general studies/ evening classes, vocational/trade/beauty schools

Work Adjustment Training, Work Hardening program, (see also section 22. Basic Work Skills), work placement, internship program

Residential Services: foster care, "group home", Community Living Arrangements, community residential services, "half-way house", structured/supportive living arrangement, transitional services, protective services, etc. (see also section 21.1 Living situation).

Note: You may want to create/insert a reference list of additional services available in your community or system.

YVONNE DAVIS

## Recommendations, Prognosis

### For a Child:
Methods and services to be provided are to include:

Special Education, Language Stimulation classroom, Socially and Emotionally Disturbed, Hearing Impaired, in-home teacher, etc.

Counseling, psychiatric consultation, behavior modification, parent-staff conference, medical consultation, due process procedures, social skill training - remedial/adaptive/ for acceptance

## 15.2 Treatment Plan:

Problem List, Problem-Oriented Record: Subjective, Objective, Assessment, Plan notes,

Objectives/goals/outcomes, methods/means/modalities, resources required, staff and others involved, frequency of contacts, expected date of achievement, dates of review

Next appointment is scheduled for ... with (professional's name/agency)

### For a Child:
Individualized Education Plan as required by Public Law 92-142, parent-staff conference

# 16. Prognosis:

PROGNOSIS FOR

> community/family/structured setting/institutional placement, for full/partial recovery, for
> competitive/supportive/partial/sheltered/workshop employment, for therapy, for life

IS

> excellent/good/uncertain because .../variable/poor/unknown/guarded/negative/grave/terminal

COURSE IS/IS EXPECTED TO BE (<->)

> benign, static, waxes and wanes, acute, shows step-wise/steady progress, recuperating, fluctuating
> with short remissions, chronic, has reached a steady state, no change with or without
> treatment, hard to treat, refractory to treatment, rapidly progressing, virulent form of the
> disorder, unrelenting course despite our best efforts, intractable, has failed all appropriate
> treatments, malignant

OTHER:

> His/her eventual prognosis for success in later life will be a function of how well the situational
> demands match his/her individual profile of abilities
> The severity and chronicity of his/her symptoms indicate a poor prognosis
> His/her history so far has been downhill and his/her prognosis therefore must be ...
> This outcome/result of treatment is expected only if (specified) services are received and is expected to
> be slow and difficult with many reversals
> S/he can be salvaged with ....
> The probable duration of treatment is __ with these (goals of therapy):

# 17. Summary

In summary/in short /to summarize...

> **For a Child:**
> His/her behavior is more like a __ year old than his/her age of __ years

MAJOR DESCRIPTIVE ELEMENTS:

This (age), (sex) (any other crucial factors) ....

HISTORY: (See section 7. Background)

FINDINGS: (select the most relevant three or four)

DIAGNOSIS: (see section 14. Diagnosis), (generally offer only the most important one or two)

TREATMENT SUMMARY:

Treatment has been a complete/partial/minimal success

S/he has followed a productive hospital course
Has received maximum benefit of treatment/hospitalization/services

Treatment received has had no success/been ineffective in removing/reducing symptoms
Treatment has had a negative outcome for this patient

PROGNOSIS: (see section 16. Prognosis)

RECOMMENDATIONS:

# 18. Closing the Report

Thank you for/I appreciate the opportunity/privilege of being able to evaluate this most interesting/
challenging/pleasant patient/person/gentleman/woman.
Thank you for allowing me to participate in his/her care/sending (patient's name) to us.
It goes without saying that I appreciate you trust in allowing me to assist in the care of this patient.
I, and my colleagues, appreciate ....

I hope this information will be useful to you as you consider this case/person/client's needs/aid you in your
tasks.
I hope this information will be sufficient for you to judge this patient's situation.
I trust that this is the information you desire/require but if it is not ....

If there are further questions I may address as a result of/on the basis of my examination of this individual
please contact my at your convenience.
I am/will make myself available for further information/consultation regarding this client's needs.
If I can be of further benefit to you in this case do not hesitate to contact me.
Please feel free to contact me if I can supplement the information in this report/if other questions or issues
arise.
If clarification is needed I can best be reached on (days) _____ from _____ to ___ (time) at (phone
number)

S/he requires no further/active/follow up from our standpoint but s/he is aware that s/he can contact us should
further problems arise.

I am/not willing to perform additional examinations/evaluations on this person.

Personal signature, degree, title

# 19. Confidentiality Notice

Attach one or more of these paragraphs to every report you send out.

This report is strictly confidential and is for the information of only the person to whom it is addressed. Any further disclosure is strictly forbidden and illegal.

Privileged and confidential patient information. Any unauthorized disclosure is a federal offense. Not to be duplicated.

This information has been disclosed to you from records protected by Federal confidentiality rules (42 CFR Part 2, P.L. 93-282) and (for example, Pennsylvania Law 7100-111-4). These regulations prohibit you from making any further disclosure of this information unless further disclosure is expressly permitted by the written consent of the person to whom it pertains or as otherwise permitted by 42 CFR Part 2. A general authorization for the release of information is NOT sufficient for this purpose. The Federal rules restrict any use of the information to criminally investigate or prosecute any alcohol or drug abuse patient.

No responsibility can be accepted if it is made available to any other person, including the person evaluated. I have in my possession a signed and valid authorization to supply these records to you and you alone.

Not to be used against the interests of the subject of this report.

Records are to be:     1. used for a stated/specific purpose, and
2. used only by the authorized recipient, and
3. not disclosed to any other party including the patient/client, and
4. destroyed after the specified use/stated need has been met.

# 20. Social Functioning

Note: If social relating has been reduced in any area try to indicate why this has happened. For sexual relating see section 5.20

## 20.1 Involvement in Activities: (<->)

Hermit, recluse, isolated, withdrawn, aloof, avoidant, no interest in social relationships, disinterested in people and relating, no social activities, keeps to self

> Doctor's etc. appointments only, no outside interests or functioning in any organizations, talks on phone, visited but does not visit, gardening and solitary pursuits, hunts/fishes

>> Window shops, visits/goes out with/drinks with friends, drops in on nearby friends, writes to or calls friends, hangs out with/ loafs with/visits family/neighbors, eats out, routine "coffee klatch"/breakfast/"night out", interested/participates in groups, small outings (church, bingo, bowling, senior center, movies), church attendance only on major holidays, friends help if s/he is sick, gets along selectively/appropriately with friends/family/authorities/public, shops in a variety of stores for all needs

>>> Gregarious, church/religious/social/card club weekly or more often, sporting events as spectator, has out of town guests, goes to movies, visits museums, musical and cultural activities, votes in elections

>>>> Attends adult school or classes, active in the community, plans life goals/self-improvement, plays team sports, visits out of town alone, does volunteer work, fully participates in the society

Note: If client reports "attends church" or "plays cards" inquire what s/he does there or which games in order to assess interests, demands (active or passive, skill or chance) and the quality and intensity of her/his social performance.

## 20.2 Conflictual Relating:

AT WORK: (see also section 22. Vocational evaluations)

> Reprimands, suspensions, firings, fighting with peers, given "cold shoulder", teases/provokes

LEGAL ASPECTS:

> Police contacts, warnings, tickets, history of fighting/drunkenness, charges filed, Protection From Abuse orders, arrests (indicate for what, when, with whom and consequences), misdemeanor, felony, trial, convictions, probation, jail/prison time, parole
> Evictions, bankruptcies
> Conflicts with neighbors, agency personnel, landlords, store clerks
> Child/spouse/relative/animal abuse

FAMILY:

> Ignored by family, distanced, never/rarely visit, only fight with, only phone contacts

## 20.3 Dating: (<->)

INTENSITY:

Never, seldom/rarely, only periodic/special events/holidays, group/car date/dyadic, "gets together with", interested in more dates but ..., frequently, has many/only brief relationships, "dating" same person for many years, many dating partners, exclusive relationship/"going steady" or "seeing others also", progressive relationships, has long-term relationships

QUALITY:

Abusive/abused, exploitative/exploited, dates compulsively, promiscuous
Satisfactory, rewarding

## 20.4 Aspects of Marriage:
Evaluate current and previous marriages.

QUALITY: (<->)

Physical/verbal/emotional abuse, abusing spouse, abused spouse, neglecting, punishing, parasitic, avoidant, 'leaky', dead, distant, stale, stalemate, "truce", unhappy, mismatched, ill-considered, hasty, unhealthy, unsupportive, limiting, unsatisfying, symbiotic, repeatedly unfaithful, stable, functional, adequate, satisfying, intimate, enhancing, loving, fulfilling

LEGAL AND SOCIAL STATUS:

Never married, (single), living together, People Of Opposite Sex Sharing Living Quarters, paramour, live-in, roommate, boyfriend/girlfriend, common-law marriage, married, separated/living apart, commuter marriage, divorced, re-married, marriage of convenience, outward appearance of a marriage

PERCEPTIONS:

Feels gets much/some/no support from spouse in parenting/child management/raising/child care, doing chores, finances, dealing with relatives, home maintenance
Child rearing is viewed as unsuccessful/overwhelming/stressful/difficult at times

## Family and Peer Relationships for a Child (see section 7.3 Personal, Family and Social History and Current Social Status/Demographics)

## 20.5 Social Maturity: (see also sections 12.11 Social maturity and 12.12 Social Judgement)

S/he is as mature as his/ her age peers, is only pseudo-mature, has been 'parentified' by his/her family, is over-mature
Never/rarely/often/usually plays/socializes with/relates to persons of his/her own age group.

Prefers to relate to things/paper/numbers/ideas/people.

# 21. <u>A</u>ctivities of <u>D</u>aily <u>L</u>iving (ADL's)

Note: If there are deficits or there has been a change indicate the reasons for this situation.

## 21.1 Living Situation/Level of Support Needed: (<->)

Lives independently in own home/apartment, uses community support services (e.g. soup kitchen, Food Bank/Community Pantry, "Meals-On-Wheels", homemaker services), with spouse/children/lover/ paramour/parental family/ relatives/ friends/roommate, single/sleeping room with/without cooking facilities, in monitored Independent Apartment, with relatives and attends Partial/Day hospital/Sheltered Workshop/Day Activities Center, in residential drug/alcohol treatment program, in rehabilitation facility, in <u>C</u>ommunity <u>L</u>iving <u>A</u>rrangement/<u>C</u>ommunity <u>R</u>ehabilitative <u>R</u>esidence/group home/supervised apartment, boarding home, custodial/domiciliary care facility, personal care home, nursing home, <u>S</u>killed <u>C</u>are <u>F</u>acility, <u>A</u>cute <u>C</u>are <u>F</u>acility, private/community/state/city/Veteran's hospital, <u>I</u>ntensive <u>C</u>are <u>U</u>nit

Note: If applicable, describe behaviors or deficits which limit independent living.

## 21.2 Self-care Skills:

Cannot feed self, assists with own feeding, feeds self, simple food preparation, bathes regularly, makeup/shaves, deodorant, grooming/haircuts, nails, hygiene, dresses self, appropriate for weather and occasion, does laundry, buys clothing, takes own medications as prescribed

## 21.3 Assistance Level: (<->)

Incapable/unable, dependent, limited only by physical/medical conditions, not psych ones, only simple tasks, directed, helps spouse/family with chores, participates, needs to be    reminded/prompted/ monitored/supervised, does with help, finishes, unassisted, initiates, independent, autonomous

ADL's done by spouse by tradition/agreement/default/because of physical limitations, ADLs performed by children/relatives/landlady/live-in friend/paid helpers/publicly provided aides

## 21.4 House Care/Chores/Domestic Skills:

Pet care, takes out trash, dishes (sets the table, clears table, washes, does pots, drys, puts away, silverware, cleans up kitchen), dusts and neatens up, runs sweeper/vacuum, straightens up bedroom, snow (shovels) and mows (grass), mops, cleans bathroom, does laundry (recognizes dirty, collects, separates, washes/runs washer, drys, folds, puts away), sewing repairs, ironing, washes windows/walls, does maintenance (changes light bulbs, recognizes malfunctioning appliances, recognizes emergencies, calls for help/repair persons), repairs (changes faucets, switches), decorates ((<->) bed covers, chooses and hangs curtains, slipcovers, paints, wallpapers), remodels

QUALITY OF PERFORMANCE: (<->)

House is immaculate/neat/clean/functional/cluttered/disorganized/chaotic/in disrepair/dangerous

## 21.5 Cooking: (<->)

Eats irregularly, eats all meals out, eats only snacks/fast-food/prepared foods/take-out/carry-out, prepares boxed-canned foods, canned soup and sandwiches, simple, top of stove, light cooking (fries, boils), full menu, nutritionally balanced, uses all kitchen appliances, coordinates foods' types and preparation times, bakes, entertains

## 21.6 Child Care: (<->)

Abuses, neglects, changesdiapers and clothes, dresses child appropriately, is affectionate with, feeds well, actively interacts with, does not leave alone, baby-sits, defends, amuses/entertains, teaches, disciplines effectively, advocates for

## 21.7 Financial: (see also section 22.4 Mathematical ability) (<->)

Not able to manage own finances, mathematically/intellectually/ emotionally incompetent, not financially competent, able to handle small sums/make own purchases/but not larger sums/checking/bill paying/saving/investing

Counts, makes change, has receptive and expressive recognition of denominations of coins/metal money/currency, handles all finances on a cash basis

Writes checks, deposits checks, able to do routine banking, saves money for large purchases, manages financial resources

## 21.8 Shops: (<->)

FOR:

Snacks, can run errands for self/others, toiletries, own clothes, simple foods, prepared foods, full menu foods, as entertainment, for presents, waits for and recognizes bargains/sales, makes major purchases

Is able to estimate the costs of common foods/items, knows which store sells which kinds of merchandise

## 21.9 Transportation: (<->)

Uses special bus, para-transit, mass transit/regular buses, driven, drives with companion, drives alone, vacations
Gets about by walking/bicycling/etc.

## 21.10 Lifestyle:

LOCATION:

Rural, farm/ranch, suburban, urban, small/medium/large city, inner-city, commuter

QUALITIES: (<->)

| | | | | | |
|---|---|---|---|---|---|
| Nomadic | Unstable | low variety | solitary | low activity | comfortable |
| vagrant | limited by | low stress | vegetative | no productive | independent |
| wanders | poverty | low intensity | occupying | activities | autonomous |
| migratory | survival | low demand | home-bound | low ambition | satisfied |
| predatory | marginal | minimal | reclusive | unproductive | ambitious |
| symbiotic | chaotic | mundane | | | adaptive |
| parasitic | | circumscribed | | | |
| roams | | constricted | | | |
| street person | | limited | | | |
| panhandles | | regressed | | | |
| | | centers around TV | | | |
| | | routine | | | |
| | | simple | | | |
| | | recumbent | | | |
| | | monotonous regularity | | | |
| | | home-based | | | |

## 21.11 Other Statements about ADLs:

Hoards items which are, in the evaluator's opinion, worthless and meaningless
Is aware of hazards such as in street crossing, dangers of gas odor, leaking water, loose wires

## 21.12 Quality of Performance: (<->)
Each area of ADL performance can be evaluated as to its independence, appropriateness and effectiveness.

Makes it worse, disorganized, ineffective, needs to be redone, unacceptable, sloppy, casual, neat, orderly, fastidious, meticulous, obsessive

## 21.13 Summary Statements:

Level of personal independence is adequate given socioeconomic status and lifestyle.
Adapted well to circumstances

S/he is intellectually and psychologically capable of performing ADLs but does not due to physical limitations/limited primarily by physical/medical circumstances

He/she is not able to care for his/her own needs and so requires _____ support services (see section 15.1 Recommendations)

# 22 Vocational/Academic Skills

## 22.1 Basic Work Skills:

ASPECTS: (<->)

Motor skills: poor coordination/good/adequate/normal dexterity/dextrous, eye-hand coordination

Shows minimal/unacceptable regard for personal attire or cleanliness/disheveled and sloppy/wears dirty clothes, needs a bath or shave, adheres to standards of non-offensive personal cleanliness, is cleanly but inappropriately dressed, appears typical of his/her community's workers in grooming/cleanliness/attire choice

Deficiencies of attention, concentration, persistence or pace, low frustration tolerance, easily dismayed, can focus and maintain attention, notices exceptions/failures, conceptualizes the problem, corrects situation/alters own behavior

Remembers locations/work procedures/instructions/rules

Makes no/few/occasional/an unacceptable number of errors which must be corrected by client/co-workers/supervisors

Productivity is minimal/below expected/equal to __ % of average/competitive worker's rate, quantity of work, he/she increased production by __ % over original measured rate

Attendance is unreliable/inadequate/minimal/spotty/deficient/adequate/as wxpected/excellent, has no/few/normal large number of unexcused absences per month, calls off, punctual on arrival/breaks/lunch hours, performs without excessive tardiness/rest periods/time off/absences/interruptions from psychological symptoms, dependable, responsible

He/she seldom communicates beyond basic ideas and often misunderstands directions/is misunderstood by peers/supervisors, can comprehend some non-concrete aspects of work situation, communication is usually understood by others, communications are clear and work relevant, has the ability to ask questions or seek assistance as needed

Response to supervision: rebels against supervision, resists supervision and is inappropriate interpersonally, often withdraws/refuses offers ofinteraction , is difficult to get along/work with, requires firm supervision, asks for unnecessary help, interacts with the general public/co-workers/supervisors without behavioral extremes/appropriately, reports appropriately to supervisor, works in small/large groups, is helpful to supervisor and peers

Emotional responsiveness on the job: he/she tends to become emotional/ angry/hurt/anxious when corrected or criticized and is unable to continue work, argues, responds angrily or inappropriately to comments, but with counseling or encouragement can remain at work site, verbally denies problems but will maintain composure and attention to task, takes corrective action, responds appropriately by adjusting behavior or work habits and shows acceptance of competitive work norms, reacts appropriately to conflict/authorities/peers/co-workers, maintains even temperament, accepts instructions/criticism/authority/supervision/feedback/ rules

Is un/able to retain individual instructions for simplest of tasks, requires constant/one-on-one supervision/continual reminders/coaching/only normal instruction to perform routine tasks, requires reinforcement to retain information from day to day, requires little or no direction after initial instruction or orientation, able to learn job duties/procedures from oral instructions/ demonstrations/written directions, carries out short/simple/detailed/multi-step instructions

# Vocational

Adaptation: "Set in his/her ways", exhibits serious adjustment problems when work environment changes, is unable to cope with job's pressures/displays inappropriate or disruptive behaviors, displays inappropriate or disruptive behavior only briefly after work changes but is able to return to task with supervisory encouragement, generally adapts to/copes with/tolerates work changes/schedules/deadlines/interruptions/pressures, relies on self, able to compete

Oblivious to/aware of hazards and able to take precautions, seems to be "accident prone" beyond usual frequency of accidents, has an "accident" whenever eligible for promotion or transfer

Cannot make simple decisions to carry out a job, indecisive, confused by choices and criteria, becomes paralyzed by decisions, makes correct routine decisions, makes up own mind, monitors own quality, has low/poor/adequate/high inspection skills, effectively sequences steps in a procedure

Cannot conform to a schedule or tolerate a full workday, performs within a schedule, sustains a routine, organizes him/herself, prioritizes work, arranges materials, shows an even work pace throughout workday, paces work, shows necessary/expected/normal/required stamina, maintains motivation, completes assignments, finishes what s/he starts, continues despite obstacles/opposition/frustrations, able to work in a time-conscious manner, conscientious worker

Maintains/cares for tools/supplies/equipment, repairs, adjusts, replaces, services, does not waste materials or damage equipment

Travels independently by public transportation or makes own arrangements to job site

## 22.2 Vocational Competence/Recommendations:

OVERALL COMPETENCE:

S/he is capable of performing substantial gainful employment at all levels.
There are no psychological barriers to employment.

Would/not be able to meet the quality standards and production norms in work commensurate with his/her intellectual level
Can perform activities commensurate with his/her residual physical/functional capabilities
Can function only in a stable setting/sheltered program, in a very adapted and supportive setting, can perform in a competitive work setting, in the open labor market

Able to understand, retain, and follow only simple, basic instructions.
This person could understand, retain and follow instructions within the implied limitations of his/her Borderline intellectual functioning/mild/moderate mental retardation.
S/he is intellectually limited but not to the extent which would prevent appropriate employment.
S/he is functional in her/his current simplified lifestyle/supportive situation but in a more independent setting, i.e. living independently/alone s/he appears to lack adequate self-direction and other resources for maintenance/continued functioning.

Requires appropriate pre-vocational experiences, Work Adjustment Training, work hardening program, diagnostic work study, evaluation of vocational potential

Can/can't tolerate pressures of workplace, unused to the regularities and demands of the world of work

No Residual Functional Capacity for Substantial Gainful Activity

The cumulative impact of the diagnoses present very significant deterrents/obstacles to employment/productivity/substantial gainful activity

SETTING NEEDED:

Non-stressful, low/non-pressured, non-competitive setting

When performing simple, basic, repetitive, routine, slow-paced/unpaced

Solitary, non-social tasks, working alone, no contact with the public

Closely supervised

Sheltered/highly supportive, stable

Part-time, flexible hours, full-time, overtime

EMPLOYMENT LEVEL: (<->)

Unskilled/helper/laborer, semi-skilled, skilled, professional, managerial, self-employed

SUPERVISION: (<->)

Requires continual re-direction, repetition of instructions, working under close and supportive supervision, instruction only, monitoring only, occasional overview, can work independently

AMBITION: (<->)

None, lethargic, indolent, listless, lackadaisical, self-satisfied, content, eager, persistent, enterprising, greedy, opportunistic, pretentious, grandiose

JOB HUNTING: (<->)

Poor/low/adequate/high knowledge of vocational and educational resources, employment is seen as too/highly/moderately/mildly/tolerably/not stressful, has a feasible vocational goal/time frame for actions, job finding skills, interviewing skills, ability to identify obstacles to successful completion of training/skill development/employment

SUMMARY OF OBSTACLES TO SUCCESS:

Academically so deficient that s/he cannot find or hold a job

Takes unscheduled breaks/absences

Engages in excessive off-task behaviors

Invents excuses for lateness/absences/mistakes/inattention, irresponsible,

Avoids some tasks, inappropriate or disruptive behaviors, agitates intentionally, asks for unnecessary supervision/help/attention

Does not work effectively when under any/normal pressure

Responds to criticism with anger/anxiety/hurt/withdrawal

Uses/overuses offensive language

Puts worst foot forward

While not disabled s/he is not employable because ...

## 22.3 Written Language Skills/Ability: (see also section 23.4 Reading Materials)

(Test with a paragraph from a magazine on a current topic and ask about its meanings)

READING COMPREHENSION:

> Alexic, illiterate, functionally illiterate, lacks basic/survival reading skills
> Names letters, says simple words, reads out-loud/silently, only small sight reading vocabulary, reads signs/directions/instructions/recipes, low/normal comprehension, deciphered word meanings, slow reader
> His/her spelling/reading is limited to a small group of memorized words.
> Worked hard, asked for assistance, recognized errors, used word attack skills to successfully identify/decipher several words on a reading test.
> He/she has rudimentary phonetic abilities but cannot identify unfamiliar or phonetically irregular words.
> Reading skills are adequate for basic literacy and utilization of written texts for getting directions.
> His/her poor reading skills prohibit responding to/guidance by written instructions.
> Basic functional literacy/no reading for pleasure/usual skills/literate/avid/scholarly

SPELLING:

> Agraphic
> Letter-sound relationships are absent/poor/good/need strengthening
> Her/his spelling skills are poor/good/excellent and s/he shows/demonstrates a solid grasp of underlying phonetic principles.
> Writing from dictation: reversals, inversions, omissions, substitutions, additions, confused attack at letters, labored writing, reckless
> Handwriting: quality, upper and lower case letters, named the letters, inversions, reversals, confused one letter with another, degree of effort required, awkward handgrip position/use of the page, size of letters
> Relationship of disorder to expected school achievement is ...
> Areas of educational strength/weakness/ handicap, diagnosis, diagnosis of learning disabilities, need for interventions

## 22.4 Math Ability: (see also section 21.7 Financial)

> Anumerate, can say the digits, knows the sequence, holds up the right number of fingers when asked for a number, counts items, does/doesn't know which number is larger

> Understands all prices, counts change, makes change.
> Possesses basic survival math (measurements, portions, percentages, fractions, weights, etc.), basic business math
> Can do simple tasks of counting and measurement but not computation beyond addition and subtraction
> Could do simple addition and subtraction of only single digit numbers/double digit numbers but only when borrowing was not involved
> His/her ability was limited to simple computation in orally presented arithmetic problems, could answer statement/verbally presented problems requiring addition/subtraction/multiplication/ division
> Could do problems when regrouping was/wasn't required.
> Could solve/not do correctly problems involving multiplication or division, decimals, fractions or measurements

## 22.5 Academic/Vocational History:

No problems with firings, absenteeism, conflict with peers/ co-workers, supervisors

(<->) Never worked/had a wage-earning job outside the home, number/duration/kind of jobs, currently employed, unemployed, laid off, underemployed, labor pool, marginal, temporary, seasonal, part-time, full time, several jobs, retired.

(<->) Regular/irregular/interrupted/sporadic employment history, number and reasons for firings

Because of genetic/home/school situations/other background s/he didn't benefit from formal education.

**Vocational**

Notes and Additions/Suggestions:

# 23. Recreational Behaviors

## 23.1 Entertainment:TV/Radio/Tapes/Records/Music: (<->)

Avoids, dislikes, confused/over-stimulated by, just as background, passive listener, aware of news/weather, selective/chooses/plans for particular programs, "Must see my stories/soaps", recalls, actively tapes/records/purchases recordings, attends musical events regularly, plays musical instrument

## 23.2 Hobbies:

No hobbies, does crafts, needle-crafts, tinkers, paints by the numbers/water/oil/acrylics, builds models, hunts/fishes, gardens, table games (cards, checkers, Monopoly), reads, collects, repairs, plans, travels, builds

Cares for pets: feeds, exercises, cleans up after, grooms, cleans, teaches, consults veterinarian, etc.

## 23.3 Sports: (specify which)

Watches on TV, attends/spectates, reads about, discusses, participates, Special Olympics, bowling league, plays on sports team, has individual sport(s), regularly participates in sport, competitive player

Exercises: regularly, walks, jogs, aerobics, health club, golfs, swims, lifts weights

## 23.4 Reading Materials: (See section 22.3 Language ability)

NEWSPAPER:

Headlines only, comics, horoscopes, simple stories, advertisements/prices, classifieds, news, columnists, editorials, news analyses, arts sections, reviews

MAGAZINES:

Word-finding magazines, children's books/magazines, comic books, adventure, gossip, supermarket, women's, men's, news-weeklies/current events, crosswords, science fiction, special interest, e.g. war/ detective/biker/guns/wrestling/hobby/trade/technical/professional/literary/arts

BOOKS:

Romances, short stories, mysteries, novels, westerns, horror, adventure, science fiction, contemporary literature, poetry, biographies, self-help, non-fiction, texts, classics

## 23.5. Summary Statements:

QUALITY OF PERFORMANCE (<->)

No recreational activities, nothing for relaxation, for fun, no pleasurable activities, no interest in recreation

Active and satisfying recreational life, recreation integrated into work and social lives

Compulsively completes, finishes, usually does, finishes only the simplest, quickest, forgets activities started, is very slow, takes much longer than usual, previously, completes only at a very low quality, neglects, half finishes projects, discontinues

# 24. Other Areas of Evaluation

## 24.1 Developmental Status

**For a Child:**

Consider development achieved, as compared to his/her age peers, in motor, cognitive, social, communication, psychological, social, interpersonal, identity areas

## 24.2 Effect of Impairment on Person:

(<->) Has become psychotic, suicidal, regressed, decompensated, devastated, catastrophic reaction, denial of event or its consequences, overwhelmed, maladaptive, deteriorating, depressed, adjustment disorder, prolonged/delayed mourning, saddened, marginal functioning, accepting, adjusting to disability/losses, adequate/fair functioning, functional, adapting, using psychological coping mechanisms, compensating, has devised compensatory/prosthetic/mnemonic devices, successful, over-compensating, mature, is challenged

The cumulative impact/effect of his/her emotional and physical impairments results in no/insignificant/mild/significant/moderate/severe/crippling limitations

## 24.3 Coping Ability/Stress Management:

DIMENSIONS:

Instrumental, affective and escape coping

COPING SKILLS: (<->) (See also section 7.6 Adjustment history)

Inept, incompetent, "can't cope", unadaptable, rigid, inflexible, stubborn

Resourceful, skilled, "survivor", courageous, realistic, adaptable, flexible, adjusts, conforms, bends

Valiant, proud, resourceful, "down on his/her luck"

Yvonne Davis

## 24.4 Competence to Manage Funds:

Assessment of Financial competence *is based on*:

Psychological/MENTAL STATUS evaluation/data base of orientation, memory, judgement, reading ability, emotional disturbance, intelligence testing

Psychological/psychiatric evaluation of quality of REALITY CONTACT because of delusions, hallucinations, thought disorder, etc.

His/her FACTUAL KNOWLEDGE of the source and extent of his/her assets, understanding of financial terms and concepts, recognition of currency, values/costs of several common items, simple/basic arithmetic, change making ability, perception of situations of potential exploitation

His/her BEHAVIOR such as observed/historical ability to conduct transactions, conserve assets, competent performance of financial management/responisbilities

And s/he is therefore considered:
incompetent in all financial areas
competent to manage only small amounts of money
able/not able to manage his/her property
likely/unlikely to dissipate/squander his/her property.
able avoid exploitation, manage welfare/etc. benefits, and make long range financial decisions autonomously, responsibly and effectively
likely/unlikely to fall victim to/become the victim of designing persons, be duped/gulled
lacks/possesses the capacity to make or communicate responsible decisions about the use and management of his/her entitlements and assets
unlikely to hoard funds rather than make necessary purchases

If benefits are awarded s/he would use the money for drugs/alcohol/gambling/disorganized/impulsive purchases and therefore s/he may/will/should not be the best recipient of funds for their management.

## 24.5 Estimate of Intelligence:

Consider levels of Adaptive Behavior, Activities of Daily Living as well as the results of intelligence testing.

Consider the potential effects of depression, dementia, distracting anxiety, relationship with the examiner, intercurrent medical illnesses, etc. on intellectual functioning.

DSM III-R CATEGORIES FOR MENTAL RETARDATION:

IQ levels as guide

| | |
|---|---|
| Borderline intellectual functioning (not MR, use V code 40.00) | 71- 84 |
| Mild retardation | 50-55 to approximately 70 |
| Moderate retardation | 35-40 to 50-55 |
| Severe retardation | 20-25 to 35-40 |
| Profound retardation | less than 20-25 |
| Unspecified mental retardation | not testable |

WECHSLER DERIVATIONAL INTELLIGENCE QUOTIENTS FOR THE WAIS-R (1981):

| | IQ scores as a guide | % of population included in each category |
|---|---|---|
| Very Superior | 130 and above | 2.2 |
| Superior | 120-129 | 6.7 |
| Bright Average | 110-119 | 16.1 |
| Average | 90-109 | 50.0 |
| Low average | 80-89 | 16.1 |
| Borderline intellectual functioning | 70-79 | 6.7 |
| Mild Retardation | 60-69 | |
| Severe retardation | 20-34 | |
| Moderate retardation | 50-59 | < 2 |
| Severe retardation | 20-34 | |
| Profound retardation | less than 20 | |

VALIDITY:

The obtained test scores are believed to be valid indicators/significantly underestimate current intellectual functioning/are consistent with developmental history and degree of functional loss but not potential because ....

Notes:

After three years from the date of the evaluation test data and findings should be treated with caution and trusted even less when the subject is/was a child.

Generally IQs below 40 are not clearly meaningful.

Consider the possibility that current functioning represents a decline due to Organic Brain Syndrome and, if so, give an estimate of premorbid intelligence based on current subtest results, earlier testing, changed levels of adaptive behavior, etc.

For reference purposes:

THE DSM II CATEGORIES FOR MENTAL RETARDATION:

| | IQ levels as guide |
|---|---|
| Dull normal | |
| Borderline intellectual functioning | 68-83 |
| Mild retardation (old usage is Moron) | 52-67 |
| Moderate retardation | 36-51 |
| Severe retardation | 20-35 |
| Profound retardation | less than 20 |

CATEGORIES OF MENTAL DEFECTIVENESS IN THE UNITED KINGDOM:

| | |
|---|---|
| Feeblemindedness | 50-90 |
| Moron | 50-75 |
| Imbecile | 25-50 |
| Idiot | less than 25 |

Each of these is qualified by *high, medium* or *low*.

## 24.6 Evaluation of Intellect:

If you suspect the presence of a learning disability, mental retardation or any physical condition which would affect school performance consultation with and referral to a school psychologist or educational specialist who can utilize the many specialized instruments for evaluation and remediation is usually appropriate. Commonly used and well standardized instruments include:

FOR PRECISE EVALUATION AN INDIVIDUAL'S INTELLIGENCE:

> The Wechsler Preschool and Primary Scale of Intelligence (WPPSI)
> The Wechsler Intelligence Scale for Children - Revised (WISC-R)
> The Wechsler Adult Intelligence Scale - Revised (WAIS-R)
> > all Wechsler test offer a Verbal Intelligence Quotient, a Performance IQ, and a Full Scale IQ
> The Stanford-Binet Intelligence Test - Form L-M, Revised (SB-LM), Fourth Edition
> Cattell Infant Intelligence Scale

FOR SCREENING OF INTELLIGENCE

> Columbia Mental Maturity Scale (CMMS)
> Peabody Picture Vocabulary Test (PPVT) - for non-verbal responders
> The Quick Test

## 24.7 Other Evaluation Instruments:

There are thousands published and hundreds with good reliability and validity for evaluation of almost any aspect of mental functioning. These are the most popular.

CHILD DEVELOPMENT/ADAPTIVE BEHAVIORS:

> Bayley Scales of Infant Development (the Bayley scales)
> Denver Developmental Screening Inventory
> The Vineland Social Maturity Scale (the Vineland)
> Normative Adaptive Behavior Checklist
> Various inventories of the adaptive behavior of specific populations.

EDUCATIONAL ABILITY AND ACHIEVEMENT:

> Illinois Test of Psycholinguistic Ability (the ITPA )
> Wide Range Achievement Test - Revised (WRAT-2R for adults, WRAT-R for children)
> Differential Ability Scales

LEARNING DISABILITIES:

> The Beery Developmental Test of Motor Integration (the Beery)
> Visual Auditory Digit Span (VADS)

VOCATIONAL GUIDANCE

> Differential Aptitude Tests
> Strong Interest Inventory
> Self-Directed Search

INTEGRATED ASSESSMENT

    System of Multicultural Pluralistic Assessment (SOMPA) - for children

NEUROPSYCHOLOGICAL FUNCTIONING:

    Halstead-Reitan Battery
    Luria-Nebraska Neuropsychological Battery
    The Bender Visual Motor Gestalt Test (Even with the Canter Interference procedure it is of much
        lower validity)

MEMORY:

    The Wechsler Memory Scale - Revised (WMS-R), and the Russell modification.
    Benton Revised Visual Retention Test

PERSONALITY:

*Objective:*

    For diagnosing clinical populations:

        Minnesota Multiphasic Personality Inventory (the MMPI)
        Psychological Screening Inventory

    For non-clinical populations:

        California Personality Inventory-Revised (CPI-R)
        Jackson Personality Inventory
        Sixteen Personality Factor test (16PF)
        Omnibus Personality Inventory (for older adolescents and young adults)
        Children's Personality Questionnaire

*Projective:* (These are of lower validity)

    Rorschach or Holtzman Inkblots
    Thematic Apperception Test (the TAT)
    Rotter Incomplete Sentences Blank
    Draw-A-Person test (DAP)
    Koppitz Human Figure Drawing Test
    House-Tree-Person (drawings) test (HTP)

NOTES AND PREFERENCES:

24.8 Major publishers and distributors of psychological tests and reference materials. Catalogs are free and these are listed alphabetically.

Consulting Psychologists Press, Inc. P.O. Box 60070, Palo Alto, CA 94306
"Testing, teaching and training materials."

Institute for Personality and Ability Testing, Inc. 1801 Woodfield Drive, Savoy, IL 61874. 1-800-225-4728
A catalog "of psychological assessment instruments, computer interpretative services, and books."

Multi-Health Systems, Inc. 908 Niagara Falls Blvd. North Tonawanda, NY 14120-2060. 1-800-666-7007
"Assessment material and computer software for mental health, education, industry, organizations, and research."

National Computer Systems, Professional Assessment Services, P.O. Box 1416, Minneapolis, MN 55440. 1-800-NCS-7271
A variety of tests and scoring systems.

PAR-Psychological Assessment Resources, Inc. P.O. Box 998, Odessa, FL 33556. 1-800-331-TEST
"Testing Resources for the Professional"

The Psychological Corporation, 555 Academic Court, San Antonio, TX 78204-2498. 1-800-228-0752
A large catalog of "tests, products, and services for psychological assessment" from the largest publisher and distributot.

PRO-ED, 8700 Shoal Creek, Austin TX 78758-6897. 512-451-3246
A large catalog specializing in special education materials.

Slosson Educational Publications, P.O. Box 280, East Aurora, NY 14052. 1-800-828-4800
Test products for all educational settings.

Western Psychological Services, 12031 Wilshire Blvd. Los Angeles, CA 90025. 1-800-222-2670
A large catalog of a major publisher of evaluation materials and books for all practice areas of psychology and counseling.

# 25. Personality Descriptors

For each syndrome there are listed descriptive words and phrases organized into clusters. No validity claims are made for the clusters or their contents, only that these descriptors are commonly used in psychological reports and in research studies (see especially Million, 1986).

It is sometimes useful to convey a client's personal style by reference to characters in the public media by do not overdo it.

These types are arranged simply in alphabetical order. Because the clusters and concepts overlap do review other similar types which are cross-referenced.

## 25.1 Aggressive Personality: (see also section 25.17 Sadistic personality)

CARDINAL FEATURES:

Aggression, low self restraint

BEHAVIORS:

Reckless, unflinching, fearless, undeterred by pain/danger/punishment, vicious, brutal, pugnacious, temperamental

INTERPERSONAL:

Competitive, intimidating, dominating, surgent, obstinate, controlling, humiliating, abusive, derisive, cold-blooded, persecutes, malicious

COGNITIONS:

Opinionated, close-minded, prejudiced, bigoted, authoritarian

SELF-IMAGE:

Proud of independence, hardheaded, tough, domineering, power-oriented

## 25.2 Antisocial Personality: (see also section 25.16 Psychopathic Personality)

CARDINAL FEATURES:

Predatory attitude and behavior toward others, long-standing indifference to, and repetitive violation of others rights.

BEHAVIORS:

Irritability and aggressiveness, impulsivity, impetuous, spur-of-the-moment, short-sighted, incautious, imprudent
History of drug/alcohol/telephone/etc, overuse and abuse, uses ruses, prevaricates

COGNITIONS:

Low insight, low planning, lack of consideration of alternatives or consequences, projects blame

AFFECTS:

Lacking in remorse/guilt/regret, insensitive, lacks compassion, hardened, callous, cold-blooded, emotionally detached, low motivation to change, easily bored

SOCIAL:

Irresponsible, untrustworthy, evades responsibility, uses guilt inductions on others, unreliable, rejects obligations, superficial relationships, ruthless
Unique and self-serving ideas of "right and wrong", a chronic pattern of infringement on the rights of others, violates social codes by lies or deceits, chronic speeders and drunk drivers,
Indifferent to the rights of others, revengeful, rebellious
Intolerance of delayed gratifications, irritable and easily provoked to violence

## For a Child:

Lying, truancy, starting fights, vandalism, tortured or abused ("played tricks on") animals/pets, early and extensive drug and alcohol use,

Cleckey's criteria modified from *The Mask of Sanity* (1976) 5th Edition, St Louis: C.V. Mosby

Considerable superficial charm, poise, calmness, verbal facility, pleasant and convincing exterior, lies/cheats/steals with poise
Unpredictable, disregard for obligations, no sense of responsibility in work, sexual, family or financial relationships
Insincerity, untruthfulness, disregard for the truth
Lack of remorse, shame, concern, anxiety
Inexplicable impulsiveness, poor planning, no inhibitions on behaviors, recklessness, almost unmotivated misdeeds, perverse quality to these behaviors
Failure to learn from experience, poor judgement
Failure to believe his/her behavior will be punished
Egocentricity, incapacity for attachment, lack of concern for others, empathy, loyalty, poverty of deep or lasting emotions, shallowness
Lack of capacity for insight or seeing oneself as others do
Ingratitude, arrogance
Impersonal, trivial and poorly integrated sex life

Anxious Personality (see 25.12 "Nervous" Personality)

Attention Deficit Disorder with and without Hyperactivity (see section 13.1 ADD with H)

## 25.3 Avoidant Personality:

CARDINAL FEATURES:

Oversensitive and vacillating, watchful for any hint of disapproval, discomfort in all social situations

INTERPERSONAL:

Yearns for closeness/warmth/affection/acceptance, but fears rejection/disapproval in relationships
Withdrawing, guarded, private, lonely
Wary, distrustful, vigilant for offenses/threats/ridicule/abuse/humiliation, hypersensitive/keen
    sensitivity to potential for rejection or humiliation by others, expects not to be loved, needs
    constant reassurance/guarantee of uncritical affection
Shy and reticent, timid, fear "goofing up"/gaffs/social errors and so "making a fool of themselves",
    fear cry/blush/embarrassment

AFFECTS:

Anguished, lonely, sad, angry, intensely ambivalent, "bored"

SELF-IMAGE:

Devalues own accomplishments, angry and depressed at self for social difficulties, sees self as
    isolated and rejected

OTHER:

Vicious cycle of low self-esteem, fear of rejection, shallow or awkward attempts at social relating,
    hypersensitivity to lack of enthusiasm/disapproval, concludes/confirms rejection, withdrawal,
    fear of relationships, loneliness, yearning, trying again, rejection, etc.
Extensive reliance on fantasizing for gratification of needs for contact and anger discharge

## 25.4 Borderline Personality:

CARDINAL FEATURES:

Instability in all aspects of living, personality functioning, mood and social relating, lack of personality consistency/cohesiveness, "cuts loose"/abrupt shifts of affect/relationships

BEHAVIORS:

Impulsiveness, sudden dramatic and unexpected outbursts, mercurial, manipulative suicide gestures or attempts/overdosing, running up huge bills/shoplifting/gambling sprees/eating binges/sexual acts, impulsivity/poor judgement, addictive traits and patterns, self destructive/mutilating/damaging behaviors

INTERPERSONAL:

Intense and unstable relationships, inexplicable changes in attitude/feelings toward others, capricious, "ups and downs", vacillating reactions, dependency-independency cycles,
Intense dislike of isolation and loneliness so engages in a series of transient/ stormy/brief relationships, superficiality of relationships based on alternating idealization and deflation

AFFECTS:

Labile, brittle, erratic, unpredictable, tenuous and shifting controls, barely hidden anger/under the surface, pessimism, argumentativeness, irritable, easily annoyed, sarcastic, intense and sudden rages or depressions, spells of emptiness and boredom, dejection and apathy, numbness
Areas of seemingly unalterable and crushing negativity, worthlessness/badness/blame/fault assumption

IDENTITY:

Shaky, shifts of identity/gender identity/career choices/long term goals, frequent "Who am I?" questions, nebulous, multiple identities/personalities, splitting, instability of self-esteem, self-image, personal and sexual identity, uncertain values, loyalties

OTHER:

Mixed picture with elements of other Personality disorders present, often affective disorder diagnoses

## 25.5 Chronic Pain Syndrome:

PAIN BEHAVIORS:

Groans, flinches, winces, grimaces, grits teeth, slow and careful movements and body placements, assumes/maintains odd positions, need to shift position/stand/walk/stretch frequently, takes multiple/ineffective medications, increased resting ("down") time and decreased active ("up") time, appears fatigued, decreased or absent sexual activity/duration/frequency/interest, decreased sleep effectiveness, interference with appetite, lessened concentration

MOOD:

Restricted range and intensity of expression, irritability, "cranky", anger, hostility, threatening, resentful of unfair way treated by helpgivers/insurance carriers, overly or disrespectful, critical, depressed, demoralized, pessimistic, expressions of hopelessness, hopeless of change/improvement/ return to work, intermittent depressions as reaction to pain's exacerbation

THOUGHT CONTENT:

Preoccupied with losses/accommodations/somatic conditions/treatments/pains/symptoms/health status and its implications, focus on small signs of progress, may create illusory correlations of pain/limitations/ depression/symptoms with progress/change/bodily processes
Feels "like a cripple", worthlessness because 'worth less', optimistically reports "learning to live with it/the pain"
Desperate for the situation to change but doubting the effectiveness of any intervention.
Has a sense of entitlement, focuses on the unfairness of the situation
Inward focus on physical self which is not hypochondrical but a reaction to chronic pain
Suicidal ideation in the form of passive death wishes

SOCIAL:

Decreased social activities/withdrawal/isolation, decreased or absent recreation
Adopts role of "patient": dependency, passivity, helplessness, avoidance/ displacement of responsibility, medical/biological model of pain and recovery, etc.
Feels/believes himself harassed/unappreciated by his current or former employer(s), or Workman's Compensation Boards/insurance companies/Social Security Disability
Reports being "sick and tired" of pursuing insurance claims, being medically evaluated, filling out forms, "jumping through hoops", to only obtain what is rightly his/hers.

OTHER:

Wants to be believed more than being relieved, concerned that his/her symptoms be accepted as authentic
Takes medication although reports its ineffectiveness/valuelessness
Seeks a "miracle cure" vs. accepts limitations and "tries it another way"

Notes: For some clarity of the evaluation of the psychogenicity of pain see Hackett's (1978) MADISON scale. He believes that pain is more likely to be psychological if the client shows: Multiplicity of varieties and places, Authenticity or need to be believed, Denial of emotional problems or of the effects of emotions on pain, Interpersonal relationships' affecting the pain, Singularity of the pain problem, "Only you" can help me, and Nothing helps or No change in the pain.

For more detailed documentation of the pain use the McGill-Melzak Pain Questionnaire in Melzak and Wall (1982) or Feurstein and Skjei (1979).

## 25.6 Compulsive Personality: (See also section 25.13 Obsessive Personality)

CARDINAL FEATURE:

Repetitious behaviors or irresistible anxiety

AFFECTS

His/her only pleasure is in elaborate planning, only mild/brief pleasure with the completion of projects, a "work" not "pleasure" orientation, perceived lack of control of environment leads to intense depression, great need and effort to control tension and anxiety, unrelaxed, joyless, solemn, grim, controls most emotions, occasional intense righteous indignation
Fears of contamination

BEHAVIORS:

Rituals of magic or checking, hoarding, highly regulated/organized lifestyle, a "checker", a "hand-washer"

COGNITION:

Rumination prevents task completion, hyper-careful, doubting, indecisive, poor decision making and follow-through, poor time management, excessively moralistic concerns, scrupulousness, intense self-evaluation/scrutiny, 'black or white' judgements
Perfectionistic approach, over-attention to detail and avoidance of error, need for immediate closure, concern with form over content/procedures/regulations more than the goal/letter of the law not the spirit/ orderly task procedures rather than the outcome, sees the world in terms of schedule/rules/regulations, neatness, meticulous, a "fanatic"

SELF-IMAGE:

Industrious, reliable, efficient, loyal, prudent/careful

INTERPERSONAL:

Demanding on others for doing thing his/her way, is seen as somber, formal, cold
Respectful, conventional, follows the proprieties, polite, correct
Shows reaction formation in positive, socially acceptable presentation of self

## 25.7 Dependent Personality: (See also section 25.20 Self-Defeating Personality)
Do not confuse with or assume masochism

CARDINAL FEATURE:

Undue dependence upon others

INTERPERSONAL:

Passive, docile, compliant, conciliatory, placates, self-sacrificing, deferring, uncompetitive
Dependent, allows others to assume responsibility for self, reliance on others to solve problems or
   achieve goals, decide on employment/friendships/child management/vacations/clothing/
   purchases, absence of independent decision making, avoids external demands and
   responsibilities, low self-reliance, low autonomy, exaggerated and unnecessary help-seeking
   behaviors
Submissive, dominated, abused, "imprisoned", exploited, secondary status, self-defeating, abused,
   tolerates partners abusive affairs/beatings/drunkenness, unable to make demands on others,
   "Niceifier", childlike, immature
Vicious cycle of dependency, abuse, proof of helplessness and worthlessness, avoidance of taking
   self-respecting or independent actions, lessened self-esteem, greater dependency, subordinates
   own needs so as to maintain protective relationships

BEHAVIORS:

General ineffectiveness but not incompetence but may demonstrate exceptional skill in some areas,
Lacking in skills/motivation for independent life

MOOD:

Hidden depression and angers, separation leads to depression, whiney, tantrums, complains, terror of
   abandonment

SELF-IMAGE:

Self derogating, belittling, martyr-like, self-sacrificing, low self-confidence, "inferiority complex",
   "stupid", humble, self-effacing, self-deprecating, inadequate, inept, fragile, hidden strengths
Devoted, loyal, sacrificing for "love"

COGNITIONS:

Believes in magical solutions to problems
Naive, gullible, unsuspicious, "Pollyanna"
Belief in salvation through love (*Amor omnia vincit*)

## 25.8 Histrionic Personality:

Current usage does not support "Hysteric", and they are not all females.

CARDINAL FEATURE:

Attention seeking through self-dramatization and exaggerated emotion

AFFECTS:

Exaggerated, labile/rapid/vivid/shallow affect, easily "overcome" with emotions, easily enthused/ disappointed/angered/excitable, theatrical/flamboyant/intensely expressed reactions, overly dramatic behaviors, creates dramatic effects, seems to be acting out a role, exaggerated and unconvincing emotionality

BEHAVIORS:

Overreacts to minor annoyances, inappropriate, affectations, affected, over-reactive, overdetermined Repeated/impulsive/dramatic/manipulative suicide gestures/attempts

COGNITIONS:

Forgetting, repression, unreflective, self-distracting, distractible
Lives in a non-factual world of experience, impressionistic perception and recollection/global/ diffuse, lacking in sharpness, non-analytical
Impressionable, susceptible to the vivid/striking or forcefully presented
Magical solutions to problematical situations, hunches, "women's intuition", child-like, does not adapt to change well
Superficial and stereotyped insights
Creative and imaginative

INTERPERSONAL:

Seductive, exhibitionistic, vain, manipulative, asserts "a women's right to change her mind", dominates conversation, trivializes topics, lengthy dramatic stories, self-dramatizing, facades, histrionic, "life of the party"/center of attention, fickle, wants to please
Romantic outlook: fantasies of rescue, nostalgia, sentimentalism, idealization of partner; world of "villains and heroes", makes poor social relationship choices and decisions, poor judgements about partners/friends/spouses
Initially seen by others as warm and affectionate, guileless, vivid. Later seen as selfish, shallow/superficial and insincere, ungenuine, inconsiderate, self-pitying, astonishment/little understanding of the implications of her or his behavior/its consequences/effects on others/destructiveness
Oppressively demanding, taking without giving, egocentric, vain, petulant, easily bored, requires excessive external stimulation, attention-seeking, help seeking, manipulates for reassurances, excessive needs for attention/praise/approval/gratification
Helpless, dependent, suggestible, uncritical, unassertive, sees assertion as rude or nasty, seen as fragile
Impetuous, period of wild acting out, irresponsibility, bar-hopping, bed-hopping/sexual promiscuity/ casual sexuality, low/poor impulse control/judgement/insight, thoughtless judgements
Self-centered, is either hurt, deserted or betrayed in all relationships, brief and superficial contrition, sees self as sensitive and vulnerable, unsubstantial sense of self, absence of political or other convictions
Stormy relationships, with little real or durable enjoyment

STYLIZED/CARICATURED "FEMININITY":

"Faints" at the sight of blood, swoons, "vapors", coy, seductive, flirtatious, sexually provocative, excessive time spent in romantic fantasies, blushes, easily embarrassed, giggles, naive, lacking in accurate sexual knowledge, seductive for help not sex, preoccupied with sex
Vain, selfish, immature, overdependent, shallow, self-dramatizing/sexy/flamboyant/dramatic clothing/hairstyle/makeup, looks/dresses like a teenager/prostitute

SELF-IMAGE:

Charming, gregarious, stimulating, playful
Sensitive to others/feelings
Selective incompetencies in areas of low importance, e.g. numbers, specifics

SOMATIC COMPLAINTS:

Vague, changeable, movable, "women's problems", complains of aging/appearance changes, feigns illness, swooning, always wrong weight, *La belle indifference* (infrequent)

## 25.9 Inadequate Personality:

CARDINAL FEATURE:

Under-responsive in all life functions, immature

SELF-IMAGE:

Intense feelings of inadequacy and inferiority

AFFECTS:

Weepy sentimentalism, involvement in melodramatic situations, over-seriousness with authority figures

INTERPERSONAL:

Underproductive in all areas: conversational initiatives, qualities of emotions, depth of relationships
Victimized or abused, taken advantage of, gullible
Passive and unaware

Yvonne Davis

## 25.10 Manipulative Personality:

CARDINAL FEATURE:

Unprincipled and deceitful in dealing with others who have something s/he wants.

BEHAVIORS:

Externalizes all blame, takes no responsibility for unfavorable outcomes
Repeated, impulsive, dramatic, self-serving suicide gestures/attempts
Evasive/indirect responses to questions, dishonest, untruthful
Connives, cheats, deceptive, fraudulent, Machievellian, unethical, unprincipled, unscrupulous,
    cavalier
Disloyal, untrustworthy, unfaithful, unscrupulous

SELF-IMAGE:

Grandiose ideas about him/herself, imposter, narcissistic

SOCIAL:

Likeable, attractive, engaging, center of attention, socially capable/ effective/charming/graceful,
Tells tall tales, flip, glib, fast, witticisms, attempts to con, puns, word plays, overabundant ideas

## 25.11 Narcissistic Personality: (see also section 25.10 Manipulative Personality, above)

CARDINAL FEATURE:

Self-centeredness

ASSOCIATED FEATURES:

Exhibitionism, craves attention

SELF-IMAGE:

Grandiose sense and fantasies of self-importance/uniqueness/entitlement, "special",
Easy loss of self esteem, "a fraud/fake", times of intense self-doubt, self-consciousness
Fantasies of continuous conquests/successes/power/admiration/beauty/love,brags of his/her talents
    and achievements, predicts great success for self, believes entitled and deserving of a high
    salary, overvalues all of his/her own achievements

INTERPERSONAL RELATIONSHIPS:

Confident, self-assured, expects to be treated as a sterling success or gifted person, hides behind a
    mask of intellectual superiority, exaggerated self-esteem easily reinforced by small evidences
    of accomplishment and easily damaged by tiny slights and oversights, compliment hunger
Fragile self-esteem, compulsive checking on other's regard, responds to criticism with rage or despair
    or cool nonchalance, may ruminate for a long time over non-threatening social situations and
    interactions
Relationships are seen entirely in terms of what others can offer, arrogant, socially insensitive,
    exploitative, resents any failure immediately and totally gratify his/her needs, demanding of
    affection/ sympathy, flattery and favors
Striking lack of empathy, indifferent to rights of others, flouts the social rules, alternates idealization
    of and arrogant contempt for friends, long history of erratic relationships, takes others for
    granted, drives people away, his/her understanding of social conventions is distorted by
    egocentrism
Heedless, reckless, neglectful, indifferent, thoughtless, tactless, selfish, ungrateful, unappreciative,
    delinquent, sloppy
Oppositional/argues with authorities/instructions/examiner/supervisor, little attention paid to work
    tasks, lies to protect ego/privileges/position, rationalizes, self deceives, distorts facts
Grandiose, cocky, intimidating, belligerent, resentful, pretentious, sarcastic, cavalier, boorish,
    bumptious, obnoxious
Conversations so circumstantial that others lose interest

AFFECTS:

Nonchalance, imperturbable, insouciant, optimistic, all unless ego damage/threats
Chronic unfocussed depression

Cognitions:

Envy
Preoccupation with own performance's value, attention getting,

## 25.12 "Nervous" Personality: (see section 10.3 Anxiety)

"High-strung", worrier, anxiety-ridden, "bad nerves", excitable, easily upset, unstable, moody, skittish, temperamental

Picky, chronically dissatisfied, carping, fault finding

Avoids/dislikes crowds, socially anxious, shy, sensitive, thin-skinned, low self-esteem, hard on him/herself

Low stress/frustration tolerance, "cracks up", "falls apart"

**For a Child:** (see section 13.1 Attention Deficit Disorder)

## 25.13 Obsessive Personality: (see also 25.6 Compulsive Personality, 13.2 Compulsions, and 13.13 Obsessions)

CARDINAL FEATURE:

Over-ideational, worries, "thinks too much"

COGNITIONS:

Indecisive, doubting, balances pro and con, ponders, ruminates, over-ideational, over-deliberateness, distrusts own judgements, fears making any mistake, rejects new ideas or data, flounders, dithers, ponders endlessly, avoids decision situations, reverses decisions, wishy-washy, vacillates

Overdependence on intellect and logic, intolerant of affects

Procrastinates, dawdles, delays, avoids, denies, ineffectiveness, most tasks important done last

Preoccupation with trivial details, over-concern with technical details, compelled attention to details, "can't see the forest for the trees", "rearranges the deck chairs on the *Titanic*", a fanatic, a stickler for details, overconscientious, gives unnecessary warnings and reminders

Preoccupation with the mechanics of efficiency such as list making/organizing/schedule making/ revising/following rules, fears loss of control

Perfectionism, scrupulousness, demandingness, rigidity, inflexibility, "never good enough", judgmental, moralistic

Tense activity, effortful, burdened, driven, suffers under deadlines, pressured, racing thoughts

Mild rituals, ritualistic interests, repeated 'incantations', magical thinking

Controlled by "Tyranny of the Shoulds" (Karen Horney), "Musterbates" (Albert Ellis), overconfidence in own will power

AFFECTS:

Isolation of affect, loss of spontaneity, stiff and formal in relating, incapable of genuine/intense pleasure in anything, ambivalences, mixed feelings, depression

Terrified of being embarrassed/humiliated, fears being found inadequate/wanting/making a mistake

INTERPERSONAL:

Proper, careful, dutiful, stilted, dogmatic, opinionated, inflexible

Uncomfortable on vacations or unstructured times

Demanding and controling, but resists other's control

## 25.14 Paranoid Personality:

CARDINAL FEATURES:

Distrust and suspiciousness

INTERPERSONAL:

Distrusts, un/mistrustful of others, over-cautious, cynical, expects mistreatment and treachery, distrusts motives of others, believes others are trying to put him at a disadvantage, suspects manipulations, distrust previous "allies", skeptical, power themes in conversations, reinforced expectations lead to isolation/enhancing distrust, exaggerating distortions resulting in delusions, and the creation of a "pseudocommunity" (Cammeron)

Vigilant, sensitive to deception, betrayal, deprecation, put-downs, listens for insulting/questioning references, hypersensitivity to criticism

Guarded, immune to correction, defensive

Hostile, belligerent, oppositional, confrontational, argumentative, stubborn, quick to take offense, easily offended, desire to vanquish/humiliate/deprecate, makes disparaging remarks, revenge fantasies, preoccupied with/desires to get even, carries grudges, schemes

Desires to remain independent, no close relationships, refusal to confide, aloof, distant, isolated, withdrawn, retreats, secretive, terror of being controlled, continuous and extreme defense of autonomy, dread of passive surrender

Made indirect references to/hinted at/ideas of reference, knowing looks, winks, oblique

Difficult, rigid, oppositional, deflects criticism onto others, recognizes no faults in self, denies responsibility or blame, blames others for all negative outcomes and frustrations, externalizes blame

Carping, hypercritical, fault finding

Arrogant, prideful, overbearing, boastful, sensational plans, grandiosity, inflated appraisal of own worth/contacts/power/knowledge, takes a superior posture, disgusted by other's weakness

Never forgives or forgets, 'chip on shoulder',

A loner unless in total control of other/group, jealous of other's status

COGNITIONS::

Projects, distorts the significance of actions and facts, loss of a sense of proportion

Rigid and repetitive searching for confirmation of suspicions/ideas of reference/personalized meanings, attends only to conforming evidence/clues, belief in own convictions of underlying truth, magnifies minor social events into confirmations of the evil intentions of others and their lying, flimsy or unfounded reasons produce intense suspicion, sensitive to slights

Vigilant for signs of trickery/exploitation/abuse, hypervigilant, constant scanning for treachery, resentful, hypersensitive, hyperalert, oversensitive to any changes/the unexpected/anything out of the ordinary, fears of surprises

AFFECTS:

Shallow emotional responses, cold and humorless, absence of tender or sentimental feelings, unemotional, restricted, enigmatic and fixed smile/smug, humorless, litigious

Edgy, rarely relaxes, tension, on guard, tense, anxious, worried, threatened, motor tension, touchy, irascible, jealous, envious, jealousy of progress of others

## Personality

SELF-IMAGE:

Bitter, overlooked, feels mistreated, taken advantage of, tricked, pushed around, abused, threatened, collects injustices, suspects being "framed/set up"
Grandiose, self-important
Rational, unemotional, careful

DELUSIONAL SYSTEM: (See also section 13.3 Delusions)

Belief in unusual or irrational ways of knowing e.g. reading the future, magical thinking, ESP
Delusions of power, status, knowledge or contact

OTHER:
Auditory hallucinations/voices which command, mock or threaten

---

## Passive Personality: (see 25.7 Dependent Personality)

---

## 25.15 Passive-Aggressive Personality:

CARDINAL FEATURE:

Intentional ineffectiveness, indirectly expressed resistance to demands of others for performance, thwarts/frustrates authority/spouse/partners/relatives

INTERPERSONAL:

Autocratic/tyrannical, demanding, manipulative, harassing, ambivalent, ruminates
Troubled/conflictual marriages
Indirect control of others without taking responsibility for actions or anger, denies/refuses open statements of resistance/maintains own "good intentions", superficially submissive

VOCATIONAL:

Intentional inefficiency that covertly conveys hostility, veiled hostility, resents control/demands. sulks, argues, complains to others/"bitches", critical of boss
Qualifies obedience with tardiness, dawdling, sloppiness, stubbornness, sabotage, "accidental" errors, procrastination, forgetfulness, incompleteness, withholding of critical information/responses/replies
Not lazy or dissatisfied with job but spotty employment record, no promotions despite ability

## 25.16 Psychopathic Personality: (see also section 25.2 Antisocial Personality)

CARDINAL FEATURE:

Repetitive socially destructive behaviors.

ILLEGAL OR IMMORAL ACTIVITIES:

Lying, stealing, swindling, cheating, conning, commission or involvement in minor or serious illegal or delinquent acts, breaking the law,

Trouble with the police/juvenile or school authorities, truancy/plays a lot of hooky, been a discipline problem/expelled/suspended from school,

Steals/vandalize/"messes up" property

Conned/manipulated/cheated people out of their money/possessions, predatory, often victimizes the easiest/weakest members of society, "white collar" criminal, "bottled up" anger

SOCIAL:

Cavalier, acting wild, slept around with people he/she didn't know very well, earned money by pandering/procuring/pimping/having sex with another person

Wandered from place to place without a home for a long time, told a lot of lies, used an alias, trouble because failed to pay his/her bills

Multiple marriages/divorces, suddenly left/hit/unfaithful to his/her spouse, seriously hurt/neglected a child

Feels or believes him/herself to be harassed/misused/victimized, resents, distrusts, suspicious, justifies behavior with lies and manipulation

VOCATIONAL:

Unstable employment: fired, ran away, quit a job impulsively/without another to start, "didn't work because he/she just didn't want to", court martialed/demoted, missed a lot of work or were late a lot and so got into trouble

AGGRESSIVENESS:

Used a weapon in a fight, convicted of a felony, served time, arrested

## 25.17 Sadistic Personality:

FEATURES:

Cruelty, demeaning/aggressive behavior pattern

Enjoys making others suffer, has lied to make others suffer, intimidates/frightens/terrorizes others to gain own wants, restricts others autonomy, uses power in harsh manner for discipline or mistreatment, embarrasses/humiliates/demeans others, brutalizes others, uses threats/violence/physical cruelty to dominate others, quickly escalates level of violence to reestablish dominance, fascinated by violence/injury/torture/weapons/martial arts, etc.

## 25.18 Schizoid Personality:

CARDINAL FEATURE:

Social remoteness and emotional constriction.

COGNITIONS:

Impoverished/barren/sterile cognitions, circuitous thinking, preoccupied with abstract and theoretical ideas, vague and obscure thought processes, unconventional cognitive approach
Intellectualizes, mechanical, attends to formal and external aspects of relationships
Excessive compulsive fantasizing, fantasies are sources of gratification and motivation, hostile flavor to fantasies
Vague and indecisive, absentminded

BEHAVIORS:

Lethargic, low vitality, lack of spontaneity, sluggish

SOCIAL:

Aloof, social isolation, no close friends, "loner", an isolate, remote, indifferent to others, solitary interests, daydreams, self-absorption, may seem "not with it", inaccessible, withdrawn, unobtrusive
Limited social skills, unresponsive, unable to form attachments, "fades into the background", peripheral roles, rarely date or only passively
Indifferent to other's praise/other's feelings/criticism, complacent, lacking in social understanding
Normal or below average work performance and achievement, unless work does not require social contact

AFFECTS:

Emotional coldness, limited capacity to relate emotionally, flat, impassive, blunted affect, emotional remoteness, absence of warm emotions toward others, no deep feelings for another, unfeeling, only weak/shallow emotions, weak erotic needs, cold, stark affects

## 25.19 Schizotypal Personality:

CARDINAL FEATURES:

Having the interpersonal difficulties of the schizoid plus eccentricities or oddness of thinking, behavior and/or perception

BEHAVIORS:

Odd, curious, bizarre, undoing of "evil" thoughts or "misdeeds"
Odd speech with vague, fuzzy, odd expressions
Odd clothing or personal style

COGNITIONS:

Magical thinking - superstitiousness, clairvoyance, telepathy, precognition, depersonalization and derealization, recurrent illusions
Autistic, ruminative, metaphorical, poorly separates personal and objective/fantasy and common realities, dissociations, depersonalizations and derealizations, sees life as empty and lacking in meaning
Sometimes paranoid ideation and style

AFFECTS:

Chronic discomfort - negative affects

INTERPERSONAL:

Suspicious, tense, wary, aloof, withdrawn, tentative relationships, gauche, eccentric, peripheral, clandestine
Dull, uninvolved, apathetic, unresponsive or obliquely reciprocating

## 25.20 Self-Defeating Personality: (See also section 25.7 Dependent Personality)

CARDINAL FEATURES:

Chooses situations which would cause him/her to suffer mistreatment, failure or disappointment
Avoids pleasurable or success experiences, does not perform sucess-producing tasks despite possessing the ability, excessive and unsolicited self-sacrifice/sacrifice induces guilt in others and then avoidance, provokes rejection by others and then feels hurt or humiliated, responds to success with depression/guilt/self-harming behaviors,
Rejects or does not pursue relationships with seemingly caring or needed/helpful (e.g. a therapist) partners, chooses unavailable partners, sees those who treat him/her well as boring or unattractive, selects relationships with abusive persons, sexually stimulated in relationships with exploitative or insensitive partners, "masochistic"

## Sociopathic Personality: (see sections 25.16 Psychopathic and 25.2 Antisocial Personality)

**Personality**

Notes and Additions/Suggestions:

# 26. References

I have endeavored to remove from *The Clinician's Thesaurus* all copyrighted material (such as questions and formats of descriptions) out of respect for the efforts of the authors of important documents such as those listed below and out of recognition that any borrowed materials whose validity had been established in one format would not necessarily be valid in any other. If, after my sincere and significant efforts, any copyrighted materials remain I apologize and explain that they entered *The Clinician's Thesaurus* by oversight and from the reports written by the consulting examiners which reports I have read to compile this manual.

Included here are many variations and specializations of the Mental Status Exam which have had the benefit of empirical evaluation.

---*DSM III-R Diagnostic and Statistical Manual*, Version three, Revised. (1987). Washington: American Psychiatric Association Press. Information at 800/368-5777

--- *Physician's desk reference.* 43rd Edition, (1989). Medical Economics Company Inc., Oradell, NJ 07649

--- *Drug interactions and side effects index.* 42nd Edition, (1988) Medical Economics Company Inc., Oradell, NJ 07649

Ables, B., Brandsma, J., and Henry, G. M. (1983). An empirical approach to the mental status examination. *Journal of Psychiatric Education, 7 (3)*, 232-239.
The Empirical Mental Status Examination

Alber, M.S., Butters, N. and Levin, J. (1979) Temporal gradients in retrograde amnesia of patients with alcoholic Korsakoff's disease. *Archives of Neurology, 36*, 211-216.
The Test of Remote Memory

Attwell, Arthur A. (1972).*The school psychologist's handbook.* Los Angeles, CA: Western Psychological Services.

Baird, J. et al. (1982). *Psychological Assessment Manual..* Bridgeville PA: Mayview State Hospital.

Endicott, J, and Spitzer, R. L. (1978) A diagnostic interview: The Schedule for Affective Disorders and Schizophrenia. *Archives of General Psychiatry, 35*, 837-844.

Erkinjunti, T., Sulkava, R., Wilkstrom, J. and Autio, L. (1987). Short Portable Mental Status Questionnaire as a screening test for dementia and delirium among the elderly. *Journal of the American Geriatrics Society, 35*, (5), 412-416.

Favier, C.M. The mental status examination-revised. In P.A. Keller and Ritt, L.G. (Eds.)*Innovations in clinical practice: A source book,* Vol 5, 279-285. Sarasota, FL: Professional Resource Exchange.

Feuerstein, M. and Skjei, E. (1979). *Mastering pain.* New York: Bantam Books.

Folstein, M. F., Folstein, S.E., and McHugh, P.R. (1975). Mini Mental State: A practical method for grading the cognitive state of patients for the clinician. *Journal of Psychiatric Research, 12*, 189-198.

Garner, D. M. and Garfinkel, P. E. (1979) The eating attitudes test: An index of the symptoms of anorexia nervosa. *Psychological Medicine, 9*, 273-279.

# References

Goldenberg, B. and Chiverton, P. (1984). Assessing behavior: The nurses's mental status exam. *Geriatric Nursing, 5* (2), 94-98.

Hackett, T. P. (1978). The pain Patient: evaluation and treatment. In Hackett, T. P. and Cassem, N. H. (Eds.) *Massachusetts General Hospital handbook of general hospital psychiatry.* St. Louis: C.V. Mosby.

Haddad, L. and Coffman, T.L. (1987). A brief neuropsychological screening examination for psycho-geriatric patients. *Clinical Gerontologist, 6* (3), 3-10.

Hays, A. (1984). The Set Test to screen mental status quickly. *Geriatric Nursing, 5* (2) 96-97.

Hersen, M. and Turner, S. (Eds.) (1985). *Diagnostic interviewing.* New York: Plenum Publishing

Hinsie, L. E. and Campbell, R. J. (1970) *Psychiatric dictionary*. New York: Oxford Press (Fourth Edition)

Jacobs, J.W., Bernhard, M.R., Delgado, A., and Strain, J.J. (1977). Screening for organic mental syndromes in the medically ill. *Annals of Internal Medicine, 86,* 40-46
The Cognitive Capacity Screening Examination

Kaufman, A.S. (1979). *Intelligent testing with the WISC*. New York, N.Y.: Wiley.

Kertez, A. (1982) *The Western Aphasia Battery.*New York: Grune and Stratton

Lefkovitz, P. M., Morrison, D.P., and Davis, H.J. (1982). The Assessment of Current Functioning Scale (ACFS). *Journal of Psychiatric Treatment and Evaluation, 4*, (3), 297-305.

Lezak, M.D. (1983). *Neuropsychological assessment.* (2nd Ed.) New York: Oxford Press

Melzak, R. and Wall, P. D. (1983). *The challenge of pain.* New York: Basic Books.

Miller, P.S., Richardson, S.J. Jyu, C.A., Lemay, J.S. et al. (1988). Association of low serum anticholinergic levels and cognitive impairment in elderly presurgical patients. *American Journal of Psychiatry, 145, (3),* 342-345
The Saskatoon Delirium Checklist

Million, T. (1986). Personality prototypes and their diagnostic criteria. In Million, T. and Klerman, G. (Eds.) *Contemporary directions in psychopathology.* New York: The Guilford Press.

Mueller, J. (1984). The mental status examination. In H.H. Goldman (Ed.) *Review of General Psychiatry*, 206-220, Los Altos, CA: Lange.

Othmer, E., Penick, E.C., and Powell, B. J. (1981). *Psychiatric Diagnostic Interview (PDI).* Los Angeles, CA: Western Psychological Services.

Overall, J. E. and Gorham, D. R. (1962). The brief psychiatric rating scale. *Psychological Reports,* 10, 799-812

Pfeiffer, E. (1975) A short, portable mental status questionnaire for the assessment of organic brain deficit in elderly patients. *Journal of Geriatric Society,* 23, 433.

Pomeroy, W. B., Flax, C. and Wheeler, C. C. (1982) *Taking a sex history: Interviewing and recording.* New York: The Free Press.

Reisberg, B., Ferris, S., deLeon, M.J. and Crook, T. (1982). The Global Deterioration Scale for assessment of primary degenerative dementia. *American Journal of Psychiatry, 139* (9), 1136-39.

Robertson, D., Rockwood, K., and Stolee, P. (1982). A short mental status questionnaire. *Canadian Journal on Aging,1* (1-2), 16-20.

Rosen, W. G. Verbal fluency in aging and dementia. *Journal of Clinical Neuropsychology, 80, 2,* 135-46

Sattler, J. M. (1988). *Assessment of children* . San Diego, CA: Jerome M. Sattler.

Shapiro, D. (1965). *Neurotic styles.* New York: Basic Books.

Sovner, R. and Hurley, A.D. (1983). The mental status examination: I Behavior, speech, and thought. *Psychiatric Aspects of Mental Retardation Newsletter, 2,* (2), 5-8.

Spitzer, R.L., Endicott, J., Mesnikoff, A., and Cohen, G. (1967-8). *Psychiatric Evaluation Form: Diagnostic Version.* New York: Biometric Research, New York Psychiatric Institute.

Strub, R.L. and Black, F.W. (1985).*The Mental Status Exam in Neurology* (Second edition). Philadelphia: F.A. Davis.

Summers, W. et al. (1983). The General Adult Inpatient Psychiatric Assessment Scale (GAIPAS). *Psychiatry Research, 10,* (3) 217-236.

Teasdale, G. and Jenvet, B. (1974). Assessment of coma and impaired consciousness. *The Lancet,* July 13, 1974, 81-83
The Glasgow Coma Scale

Terman, L. M. and Merrill, M. A. (1960). *Stanford-Binet Intelligence Scale: Manual for the third revised edition* . Boston: Houghton Mifflin Company.

Wechsler, D. (1987).*Manual for the Wechsler Memory Scale - Revised.* New York: The Psychological Corporation.

Whelihan, W., Lesher, E.L., and Kleban, M.H. (1984). Mental status and memory assessment as predictors of dementia. *Journal of Gerontology, 39 ,* (5), 572-76
The Extended Mental Status Questionnaire

# Index

# Index

Response to supervision 135
Response to the methods of
    evaluation/ 73
Rituals 106
Ruminations 112

Sadistic personality 163
Schedule 136
Schizoid personality 164
Schizotypal personality 165
Schneiderian delusions 107
Schooling 52
Second-rank delusions 107
Self-care skills 131
Self-centeredness 102
Self-criticalness 89
Self-defeating personality 165
Self-deprecation 28
Self-esteem 80
Self-image 21, 80
Self-sufficiency 46
Sense of humor 92
Serial Sevens 18
Setting 137
Sexual abuse 23
Sexual adjustment 55
Sexual history 33, 52
Sexual identity 35
Sexuality 91
Shame 92
Shopping 133
Short-term retention 14
Signs 23
Similarities 17
Sleep 36
Sleep disturbances 113
Social adjustment 55
Social functioning 28, 129
Social histories 50
Social Judgement 20
Social maturity 102, 130
Social presentation 79
Social sophistication 79
Somatic/hypochondriacal 27
Somatic/vegetative symptoms
    28
Speech, amount 64
Speech behavior 64
Spelling 138
Sports 141
Station 63
Strategy 73
Stream of thought 99
Stress management 143
Stress tolerance 113

Substance abuse 37, 114
Suicidal behavior 41
Suicidal ideation 28, 115

Summary 126
Surgency 79
Symptomatic movements 62
Symptoms 23
Syndromes 23

Tardive dyskinesia 108
Task persistence 98
Test judgement 103
Thought content 94
Thought continuity 94
Transsexuality 35
Treatment plan 124
Treatment recommendations
    123
Trustworthiness 48
Truthful 48
Typical problems of children at
    home 54
Typical problems of children at
    school 53
'Tyranny of the Shoulds' 160

Uncoordinated 61

V Codes 121
Validity 48
Vegetative signs 87
Violence 110
Vocational 135
Vocational guidance 146
Voice 64
Voluntary consent 47

Warmth 80
Wechsler Derivational
Intelligence Quotients 145
Wechsler Memory Scale -
Revised 13
Witzelsucht 90

Word salad 100
Written language skills 138

# *THERAPISTS ...*

## EXPERIENCED:

Have you let your practice get too casual? Are you being careless in the litigious and watchful world we now work in?

**You know you should (but you don't):**

1. Give your patients all the Rules of Your Practice *in writing:* Here are four quite different ways to get fully informed consent to all aspects of treatment: fees, all aspects of health insurance, missed appointments, contacting you in an emergency, etc.

2. Get permission and a name for Duty to Warn if it should ever become necessary.

3. Use legally correct Collection letters and calls.

With this book you can compare your methods with what are the currently expected community standards of practice and then easily modify your practices, as necessary.

Besides those listed at right this book also offers guidelines and sources for computerizing your office.

## STARTING OUT:

Thinking of going into private practice or just getting your feet wet? Then Start Out Right! *The Paper Office* contains all the procedures and administrative forms you'll need to operate a small therapy practice legally, ethically and effectively.

1. The World's Simplest Billing Form - 20 patients in One Hour a month.

2. An "Information for Clients" brochure that covers EVERYTHING they need to know and documents it in writing.

3. Release of Information forms (FROM you, TO you, TO a lawyer, etc) which meet current legal and ethical guidelines.

4. Intake, Financial, Personal History , and Developmental  information forms.

5. Simple rules for malpractice prevention in therapy, testing and billing.

... and dozens more forms, letters and procedures with many pages of sage advice.

Now you can have all the non-clinical forms you need for the small therapy office in one 300 page book ...

# *The Paper Office*

## WHY BUY <u>OUR</u> FORMS? HERE ARE 10 GOOD REASONS

The forms in *The Paper Office* are:

1. ETHICALLY CORRECT -  They conform to current guidelines for record keeping, professional and speciality listings, confidentiality, informed consent, etc.
2. LEGALLY CORRECT - They meet government standards and current practices in the field.
3. CHEAP - It would take you many hours to design each yet you can buy all of them for less than one hour of your paid time.
4. FUNCTIONAL - They have been tested and modified over years and settings so that you can fit your practice perfectly.
5. EFFICIENT - Well integrated they require the minimum of rewriting/reentering of data yet collect all the essential information.
6. EFFECTIVE - Designed to meet insurance companies' needs, and your own needs to document diagnoses, service, progress, problems and decisions.
7. PRACTICAL - Simply and cheaply reproducible on a plain-paper copier in your office.
8. ADAPTABLE - Easily modified to fit changes in your practice (a new phone number, staff members or additional degrees or credentials) and customizeable to fit a new professional speciality or setting.
9. FRUGAL - You can make only as many as you need so there is no tossing out of hundreds of pages when you change some aspect of your practice,
10. WELL-DESIGNED - Their  handsome format enhances your professional image to clients, peers, and referral sources.

Just $39.95 plus $3.55 for shipping to *Three Wishes Press,* Post Office Box 81033, Pittsburgh, PA 15217.    *Thanks*

# 29. Feedback and Order Form          2nd Edition/3rd Printing

Dear Fellow Clinician,

I created this book to meet my needs as a clinician writing reports and gave it my best shot. I really would appreciate your best shot too so it may develop to aid all of us. New versions will come out at intervals (the next is planned for early 1992) and could be designed to better meet our needs if we work together. If you will send your suggestions, modifications and ideas (perhaps by photocopying the relevant pages) I will give you credit in the revised editions and I will send you a FREE copy of the next edition. Also if you want another or later copy of *The Clinician's Thesaurus.* there is an offer below, which you can take advantage of if you will give me some feedback on this page. Thanks.

Ed Zuckerman

Would you answer a few questions for me so I can better understand you professional life, please?

Your Professional Title: _____ Years in practice when you bought this book ___ .

How often do you refer to this book?          ❑ Whenever I evaluate people.  ❑ Every time I write a report.

❑ Fairly often, when I need some specific ideas and wording choices.  ❑ Never now; but it was useful when I was learning to write reports. Other times: _____ .

How do you use it?   ❑ I use it for questions in evaluating people.   ❑ I use it to structure my report writing.

❑ I refer to it for specific information and wording choices.  ❑ I use it to teach evaluation or report writing. Some other use(s)?: _____

What is your overall evaluation of *The Clinician's Thesaurus* in just a few words? _____

_____

I would suggest the following changes.

Increase the _____

Add the following sections _____

Decrease or eliminate _____

As a clinician I really wish there were a "tool" to: _____

We at *Three Wishes Press* are always interested in other "Tools" for clinicians. If you are developing something please write and let's talk.

❑ The Current (2nd/3rd Printing) Edition - $19.95 plus shipping and handling of $3.55 = $23.50 for new purchasers or

❑ The Current Edition if you bought any earlier edition - $9.95 and the front cover from your copy (There is, of course, a limit of one copy). The Third Edition will probably appear after 3/92 and be 15% larger.

❑ For inservice training or graduate programs, eleven copies copies sent to one address are discounted 25%.

Please make your check to Three Wishes Press, FB and send it with this page with the questions answered and your name and full mailing address to P. O. Box 81033, Pittsburgh, PA 15217. (412) 521-1057 Phone and Fax.

IF YOU ARE IN PRIVATE PRACTICE YOU REALLY SHOULD CONSIDER USING *THE PAPER OFFICE*. PLEASE SEE THE PREVIOUS PAGE.

Yvonne Davis